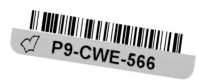

Nursing and Addictions

Editor

ALBERT RUNDIO Jr

NURSING CLINICS
OF NORTH AMERICA

www.nursing.theclinics.com

Consulting Editor
STEPHEN D. KRAU

September 2013 • Volume 48 • Number 3

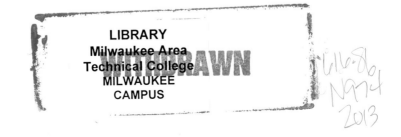

ELSEVIER

1600 John F. Kennedy Boulevard • Suite 1800 • Philadelphia, Pennsylvania, 19103-2899

http://www.theclinics.com

NURSING CLINICS OF NORTH AMERICA Volume 48, Number 3
September 2013 ISSN 0029-6465, ISBN-13: 978-0-323-18862-3

Editor: Katie Saunders
Developmental Editor: Stephanie Carter

Nursing Clinics of North America (ISSN 0029-6465) is published quarterly by Elsevier Inc., 360 Park Avenue South, New York, NY 10010-1710. Months of issue are March, June, September, and December. Periodicals postage paid at New York, NY and additional mailing offices. Subscription price per year is, $144.00 (US individuals), $374.00 (US institutions), $260.00 (international individuals), $456.00 (international institutions), $210.00 (Canadian individuals), $456.00 (Canadian institutions), $79.00 (US students), and $129.00 (international students). To receive student/resident rate, orders must be accompanied by name of affiliated institution, date of term, and the signature of program/residency coordinator on institution letterhead. Orders will be billed at individual rate until proof of status is received. Foreign air speed delivery is included in all *Clinics* subscription prices. All prices are subject to change without notice. **POSTMASTER:** Send address changes to *Nursing Clinics*, Elsevier Health Sciences Division, Subscription Customer Service, 3251 Riverport Lane, Maryland Heights, MO 63043. **Customer Service: Telephone: 1-800-654-2452** (U.S. and Canada); **1-314-447-8871 (outside U.S. and Canada). Fax: 1-314-447-8029. E-mail: journalscustomerservice-usa@elsevier.com** (for print support) and **journalsonlinesupport-usa@elsevier.com** (for online support).

Nursing Clinics of North America is covered in *EMBASE/Excerpta Medica, MEDLINE/PubMed (Index Medicus), Social Sciences Citation Index, Current Contents, ASCA, Cumulative Index to Nursing, RNdex Top 100,* and Allied Health Literature and International Nursing Index (INI).

Printed in the United States of America.

Contributors

CONSULTING EDITOR

STEPHEN D. KRAU, PhD, RN, CNE
Associate Professor, Vanderbilt University School of Nursing, South Nashville, Tennessee

EDITOR

ALBERT RUNDIO Jr, PhD, DNP, RN, APRN, CARN-AP, NEA-BC
Associate Dean for Post-Licensure Nursing Programs & CNE, College of Nursing & Health Professions, Drexel University, Philadelphia, Pennsylvania; President, International Nurses Society on Addictions, Lenexa, Kansas; Nurse Practitioner, Medical Staff, Lighthouse at Mays Landing, Mays Landing, New Jersey

AUTHORS

KATHLEEN BRADBURY-GOLAS, DNP, RN, NP-C, ACNS-BC
Assistant Professor, Graduate Nursing, Felician College, Lodi, New Jersey; Family Nurse Practitioner, Virtua Atlantic Shore Family Practice, Northfield, New Jersey

DEBORAH S. FINNELL, DNS, RN, PMHNP-BC, CARN-AP, FAAN
School of Nursing, Johns Hopkins University, Baltimore, Maryland; VA Center for Integrated Healthcare, VA Western New York Healthcare System, East Amherst, New York

GRETCHEN HOPE MILLER HEERY, FNP, BC, DrNP(c)
Lehighton, Pennsylvania

SANDRA N. JONES, DrNP, APRN, PMHCNS-BC
Doctoral Nursing Candidate, College of Nursing and Health Professions, Drexel University, Philadelphia, Pennsylvania

WILLIAM J. LORMAN, PhD, MSN, PMHNP-BC, CARN-AP
Vice President for Clinical Services, Livengrin Foundation, Inc, Bensalem; Clinical Assistant Professor, Drexel University College of Nursing & Health Professions, Philadelphia, Pennsylvania

DANA MURPHY-PARKER, MS, CRNP, PMHNP-BC
Assistant Clinical Professor; Director, Psychiatric/Mental Health Nurse Practitioner Program, College of Nursing and Health Professions, Philadelphia, Pennsylvania

SHAHRZAD NOWZARI, BS, RN
University at Buffalo, The State University of New York, Amherst, New York

ALBERT RUNDIO Jr, PhD, DNP, RN, APRN, CARN-AP, NEA-BC
Associate Dean for Post-Licensure Nursing Programs & CNE, College of Nursing & Health Professions, Drexel University, Philadelphia, Pennsylvania; President, International Nurses Society on Addictions, Lenexa, Kansas; Nurse Practitioner, Medical Staff, Lighthouse at Mays Landing, Mays Landing, New Jersey

JAMIE SMITH, MSN, RN, CCRN
Director of Practice and Education, New Jersey State Nurses Association, Trenton, New Jersey

ROBERTA L. WAITE, EdD, APRN, CNS-BC, FAAN
Associate Professor of Nursing & Assistant Dean of Faculty Integration and Evaluation of Community Programs; Interdisciplinary Research Unit, Doctoral Nursing Department, College of Nursing and Health Professions, Drexel University, Philadelphia, Pennsylvania

Contents

The role of advanced practice nursing in addictions is inclusive of the medical detoxification of patients. Addiction fits a biopsychosocial/spiritual disease model. One of the primary goals of treatment is to address the components of this model. Various pharmacologic agents have been used for the management of withdrawal.

Recovery is a continuous, progressive process of improvement whereby a person with a substance use disorder first becomes sober and then begins a lifelong commitment to improve his or her health, live a self-directed life, and strive to reach full potential. The nurse plays an important role in the beginning stages of this process by helping the patient identify relapse risk factors along with providing psychoeducational, psychotherapeutic, and psychopharmacologic interventions to decrease the risk of relapse and direct the patient down a path of self-efficacy, personal health, and productive citizenship.

The addiction to narcotic substances is an increasing public health problem. Addiction relapse is preventable. Photovoice may increase the success rate by offering a deeper perspective, insight, dimension of feeling, and perception connecting with those who feel disconnected. This process uses cameras, discussion groups, storyboards, and interaction to thread through difficult discussion points created by the participant. Understanding the process of recovery from opioid substance abuse creates an opportunity to maintain socially acceptable behaviors and decreases the risk of participating in illegal activities and making poor choices. Photovoice allows for creative expression of thought by bypassing cognitive defenses.

Addictions can be prevalent in the health professions, as these individuals are intelligent and know how drugs function. Health professionals generally also have easy access to medications and controlled substances. Many systems have been implemented in attempts to prevent nurses and other providers from abusing drugs; for example, computerized automated delivery systems of medication. Nevertheless, substance-use disorders are still prevalent in the health professions, and one cannot exclude these professionals from any discussion on substance use. This article discusses the implementation of peer-assistance programs that help nurses who abuse substances to receive treatment and maintain their licensure.

> As many as 6% to 8% of nurses are estimated to abuse alcohol or other substances. Monitoring and peer-assistance programs have been created to increase the understanding of abuse, to support nurses during their recovery and safe return to practice, and to protect public safety. In New Jersey, 2 such programs now exist: the Recovery and Monitoring Program (RAMP) and the Peer Assistance Program.

> Opiate dependency is a medical disorder that requires treatment intervention. Primary health care not only entails treatment of illness but also involves disease prevention and health promotion. Based on Pender's revised Health Promotion Model, a descriptive study comparing the health promoting behaviors/practices in abusing and recovering opiate-dependent drug users is analyzed. Using the Health Promoting Lifestyle Profile II, a comparative descriptive, exploratory, nonexperimental design study was conducted to identify key health-promoting behaviors in recovering opiate-dependent drug users. Prevention strategy recommendations are discussed, along with future research recommendations.

> With the prevalence of addiction-related health consequences, all nurses must maintain a basic level of knowledge and skills regarding addictions. Nurses are ideally positioned to screen, assess, refer; and, at the advanced practice level, treat clients for addiction disorders, provided the knowledge and willingness exists to intervene. A vision for nursing education is to achieve minimal competencies for all generalist nurses, facilitated by incorporation of substance-related disorder concepts into nursing education. An urgent need exists to disseminate the most recent knowledge and skills in nursing school curricula throughout the United States and internationally.

NURSING CLINICS OF NORTH AMERICA

RELATED INTEREST

Psychiatric Clinics of North America, June 2012
Addiction
Itai Danovitch and John J. Mariani, *Editors*

DOWNLOAD
Free App!

Review Articles
THE CLINICS

NOW AVAILABLE FOR YOUR iPhone and iPad

Preface

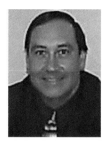

Albert Rundio Jr, PhD, DNP, RN, APRN, CARN-AP, NEA-BC
Editor

Addictions affects individuals of all walks of life. I was first exposed to addictions when I was working as an orderly in an acute care hospital's emergency department in southern New Jersey. Following completion of nursing school, I was further exposed to addictions as an emergency nurse. My first management position was an emergency department supervisor in an urban emergency department. Here is where I really became more familiar with addictions and the effects on individuals' and others' lives. I really did not understand the disease at that time. I knew it was a disease, but that was about it. My role in the hospital's emergency department was to make certain that individuals were stable medically; fed; clean; and had medical clearance for referral to a treatment center. Once medical clearance was obtained, I would then consult two of my nurses, who were in recovery, so that they could get the patient to a treatment center.

When I reflect on my experiences in the emergency department, I realize that we treated many patients for their primary symptom, such as gastrointestinal distress, and probably missed the fact that the patient's gastrointestinal distress was secondary to alcohol abuse. Now that I am so tuned, and, of course, much better educated in the disease process, I recognize the myriad of illnesses that are caused by addictions, but that a lot of clinicians miss. Many patients treated in emergency departments really have an addictions problem that was missed by the providers.

I really began to understand the disease process better when I was a Vice President of Nursing/CNO in an acute care hospital. The hospital had opened a short stay addictions unit 2 months prior to my assuming this role. I developed a very close working relationship with the medical director of the addictions unit. We had transformed this unit into a service that generated the largest number of admissions to the hospital for 11 years. I did not realize it then, but when I reflect on this, the numbers themselves demonstrate that addictions is a big problem in the United States.

I further understood the disease when I moonlighted in a correctional health setting as a nurse practitioner. The medical director of the addictions unit in the hospital had been awarded the county jail contract for the provision of medical services. He requested me to work around 10 hours per week in the jail. I saw addictions and the

http://dx.doi.org/10.1016/j.cnur.2013.08.001
0029-6465/13/$ – see front matter © 2013 Published by Elsevier Inc.
nursing.theclinics.com

treatment of such in a much different way than the hospital setting. This practice experience was life-altering for me.

My real immersion and understanding began 16 years ago when I took a part-time job as a nurse practitioner in a residential addictions treatment center that treats both adolescent and adult patients. The medical director, my collaborating physician at this facility, has taught me a tremendous amount about addictions. The nursing staff and staff in recovery have also contributed to my learning about addictions.

In 2005 I made the decision to focus my career on administration, education, and addictions nursing. This led to my involvement in the International Society of Nurses on Addictions. I was installed as the President of this organization in September of 2012.

From my work in this field, I have come to understand that addictions is a disease that crosses all walks of life. The disease has no regard for economic status, educational achievement, gender, race, creed, or nationality. I also have realized that addictions is costing society billions of dollars annually. I also realize that more of our youth are becoming addicted and one of the wars that we as providers are waging is the abuse of prescription painkillers.

What I love about this field are the patients. So many patients have been shunned and discriminated by this illness. I treat all of my patients with human dignity and respect. I learn from each and every patient and I value the fact and feel privileged that they let me into their lives to try to help them on the road to recovery.

When I was requested to be the guest editor for this issue of *Nursing Clinics of North America*, I readily accepted the challenge. My goal in this edition is to share with the reader some current information about addictions and addictions nursing. It is a very exciting time to be working in this field. We have many wonderful authors, who have written articles that focus on current information in the field. One of my goals is that you gain a better understanding of addictions and addictions nursing. Another goal is that you are able to take the information learned from this edition and apply it to your practice. We recognize that addictions crosses all practice settings. And my final goal is that you continue to educate yourself on addictions and addictions nursing. Last, I hope that many of you reading this edition decide to make addictions nursing your career. It is one of the most rewarding practices that a nurse can discover.

Albert Rundio Jr, PhD, DNP, RN, APRN, CARN-AP, NEA-BC
College of Nursing & Health Professions
Drexel University
1505 Race Street, Room 429
Philadelphia, PA 19102, USA

E-mail address:
aar27@drexel.edu

Providing Information About the Neurobiology of Alcohol Use Disorders to Close the 'Referral to Treatment Gap'

Deborah S. Finnell, DNS, RN, PMHNP-BC, CARN-AP, FAAN[a],*,
Shahrzad Nowzari, BS, RN[b]

KEYWORDS

- Screening • Brief intervention • Referral to treatment • Alcohol disorders
- Neurobiology • Health information

KEY POINTS

- About 7% of individuals who could benefit from alcohol treatment actually receive it.
- Disseminating the neuroscience behind alcohol disorders to these at-risk individuals may reduce barriers to acceptance of referral to specialty alcohol treatment.
- Nurses can integrate information about the neurobiological base of alcohol disorders in their conversations with these at-risk individuals.
- Research is needed to evaluate the impact of providing this information on acceptance of referral to treatment, engagement in treatment, completion of treatment, and long-term sustained recovery.

INTRODUCTION

Undetected and untreated alcohol use disorders are common and complicate the effective management of other health conditions. According to the Centers for Disease Control and Prevention,[1] alcohol-attributable deaths are associated with more than 35 chronic health problems and 19 acute problems. Alcohol consumption contributes substantially to the global burden of disease and has been identified as an important risk factor for premature mortality, disability, and loss of health.[2] Nurses, across all specialties, settings, and populations, are in key positions to engage patients in conversations about alcohol use, but may not view this activity as part of their role and responsibility.[3] By engaging in these patient-centered discussions, nurses can not

[a] School of Nursing, Johns Hopkins University, 525 N Wolfe street, Baltimore, MD 21205, USA;
[b] School of Nursing, University at Buffalo, 3435 Main Street, Buffalo, NY 14214, USA
* Corresponding author.
E-mail address: dfinnel1@jhu.edu

Nurs Clin N Am 48 (2013) 373–383
http://dx.doi.org/10.1016/j.cnur.2013.04.004   nursing.theclinics.com
0029-6465/13/$ – see front matter © 2013 Elsevier Inc. All rights reserved.

only respond to the call from the Institute of Medicine for nurses to practice to the full extent of their education[4] but they can also effect better care and better health and help decrease the societal cost of excessive alcohol use in the nation.

The total volume of alcohol consumed (quantity) and the pattern of alcohol consumption place people at risk. The World Health Organization has identified 4 general patterns of alcohol use: abstainers, low-risk, high-risk, and probable alcohol dependence, with 40%, 35%, 20%, and 5% of the population fitting into each category, respectively.[5] This article focuses on those individuals who are at the highest risk of experiencing alcohol-related problems with their health, work, and family—those with alcohol dependence. The human and economic costs associated with alcohol abuse and dependence command attention. In the United States for 2006, the most recent year for which data were available, the financial impact of excessive alcohol consumption was $223.5 billion or $746 per capita.[6] A further concern is that few people who need alcohol treatment actually receive it.

Data averaged across 3 annual National Surveys on Drug Use and Health found that about 8% of persons aged 12 or older (18.2 million) met the criteria for alcohol abuse or dependence in the past year.[7–9] Nevertheless, of those who need treatment, 87.4% did not receive treatment and did not perceive a need for it.[10] Among those who do perceive a need for treatment, only 1 of 7 accessed specialty substance use disorders treatment in a 3-year period.[11] Individuals who needed but did not receive alcohol treatment and who felt the need for it were surveyed to identify reasons for not receiving treatment. The most common reason given for not receiving alcohol treatment among those who felt the need for it was not being ready to stop using alcohol (42%); in addition, social stigma was also identified as a barrier.[10] Pessimistic attitudes toward the effectiveness of treatment and attitudinal factors, such as self-reliance and minimizing the problem, have also been identified as barriers to seeking treatment.[11]

What can nurses do to remove these barriers? Mojtabai and Crum[11] suggest that efforts should be directed toward improving problem recognition by the affected individuals and conveying information on the benefits of treatment for substance use disorders. This 4-part article provides a tangible way that nurses, guided by a set of clinical strategies (ie, screening, brief intervention, and referral to treatment), can be instrumental in reducing these high-risk individuals' doubts about treatment and shift their paradigm from one of self-blame to self-management by understanding the neurobiological bases for alcohol abuse/dependence and behavioral and pharmacologic treatments.

1. A brief review of the *neurobiological base for alcohol use disorders and treatments* is provided as the context for information that can and should be disseminated to this high-risk population.
2. *Clinical strategies for identifying and managing alcohol problems* are presented, which can and should be an integral part of the standards of practice for nursing.
3. An example of *disseminating neurobiological information as a brief intervention* is provided.
4. An appeal is made for studies that assess *outcomes of providing health information* as a brief intervention for this population. Research is needed to evaluate the impact of this intervention on motivational readiness to accept referral to treatment, engagement in alcohol treatment, completion of alcohol treatment, and long-term sustained recovery.

The neuroscience, related to the impact of alcohol on the brain and how the brain recovers by abstinence from alcohol, is complex. However, if that science remains in the "lab," it will not reach the "bedside." Nurses have the ability to educate and activate patients while keeping interactions short and targeted.[12] Health teaching and health promotion, among all other standards of practice for nursing,[13] are in keeping with the role of the registered nurse relative to caring for patients who are at risk for physical and/or psychological problems because of alcohol use.[3]

THE NEUROBIOLOGICAL BASE FOR ALCOHOL USE DISORDERS AND TREATMENTS

The human brain has an average of 86 billion neurons[14] with an average of 7000 connections each.[15] These cells of the nervous system are organized into circuits that process information and, in turn, give rise to our emotions, cognitions, and behaviors. The consumption of alcohol produces a wide range of effects on both excitatory and inhibitory systems in the brain, which combine to produce the characteristic mood elevating, anxiolytic, sedative, and ataxic effects of ethanol.[16] However, underlying the neurobiological basis of alcohol disorders is the brain reward system.

A chain of events is set in place when alcohol is consumed, triggered by the release of the neurotransmitter, dopamine.[17] Stored deep in the center of the brain, dopamine is associated with pleasure and euphoria.[18] Thus, these feelings, often referred to as the "high" that accompanies alcohol consumption, arise from the brain chemistry.

The flood of dopamine stimulates neurons that extend to the frontal cortex of the brain, the area lying behind the forehead. Collectively, this constellation of brain components is known as the brain reward system, an important discovery by Olds in 1954.[19] The brain reward pathway begins in the limbic brain, which is located in the center of the brain. Different components make up the limbic brain that control basic life functions, such as breathing, regulation of body temperature, and heartbeat. These functions are automatic and do not require conscious thought. The reward pathway starts in the ventral tegmental area where dopamine is produced and released. In turn, dopamine stimulates the nucleus accumbens, an area associated with motivated or goal-directed behavior. The neural pathway extends to the frontal cortex of the brain, the area of the brain associated with reasoning, cognition, and problem-solving. Understanding the brain reward system helps to explain the intense pleasure that accompanies alcohol consumption (or the reward) and attributing value to predicted outcomes of behavior.[17]

The brain is capable of change through remodeling neurons and their connections. That is, the cells can reorganize to adapt to the changing environment. This phenomenon is known as neuroplasticity, whereby the brain is able to compensate and adjust its activities in response to alcohol consumption.[20] Through this compensation, the brain is storing memories of the pleasurable feelings that result from alcohol use and structuring it in such a way as to anticipate the re-experience of that euphoria. Because these changes are unconscious, return to alcohol use can be triggered by seeing an alcoholic beverage, walking past a location where alcohol is available, hearing a song that is associated with memories of drinking, or distress, such as anxiety or stressful events. Without conscious awareness, a maladaptive pattern of alcohol use, leading to clinically significant impairment or distress,[21] begins to develop despite the consequences. Thus, the brain's neuronal circuits necessary for insight, reward, motivation, and social behaviors are co-opted,[22] explaining the "choice" to drink despite awareness of the negative consequences.[23]

The good news is that the brain is capable of recovery after a person stops drinking alcohol. Potenza and colleagues[24] describe the targets of major behavioral and pharmacologic treatments for addictions. Many, although not all, individuals with alcohol dependence, may require medical detoxification to withdraw from alcohol safely. During the initial recovery phase, the early remodeling of neural circuitry is beginning.

Although the neurobiochemical mechanisms of craving are complex and not completely understood, several neurotransmitters, such as dopamine, γ-aminobutyric acid, opioids, glutamate, and serotonin, are implicated.[25] Pharmacologic agents, such as naltrexone and acamprosate, have specific actions at certain neurotransmitters that in turn modulate dopamine function. In turn, there is a decrease in the intensity of the cravings or in the pleasurable response when alcohol is consumed.[26]

Behavioral treatments, alone or in combination with medications, have been found to be effective. Behavioral treatments focus on changing the ways one feels, thinks, and behaves when attempting to abstain from alcohol and sustain that behavior. The executive functioning of the prefrontal cortex is important in cognitive behavioral therapies, which are used to help the individual recognize behavioral patterns and cognitions that maintain alcohol use, learn, and then implement skills and strategies to effect behavior change.[27–29] Although the neural mechanisms of these behavioral treatments are not known, Potenza[24(p697)] suggests that "processes involving the receipt of health-related information and recommendations from a health professional may prompt individuals to alter their decision-making processes to focus on more future-oriented goals." The brain reward pathway is thus targeted by pharmacologic agents, which have their primary effect on the ventral tegmental area and nucleus accumbens, and by behavioral treatments that target the prefrontal cortex.

Mutual help groups provide a setting in which people can share their experience, strength, and hope freely. Because acute and chronic alcohol use affects the limbic-hypothalamic-pituitary axis,[30] as does the process of alcohol withdrawal,[31,32] the safe and supportive environment of these mutual help groups may mediate the fear that people with alcohol disorders have about being judged, blamed, or otherwise held to be personally responsible. The moral stigma was rational for the anonymity of Alcoholics Anonymous. Through interactions with others who share a similar problem, individuals have the opportunity to think about what is happening around them and to plan and organize how they need to accommodate and cooperate with others. These activities, using the frontal cortex, may help strengthen and build neural pathways, especially if this occurs within a safe setting of mutual help groups such as Alcoholics Anonymous.

Despite an abundance of science on this brain-based disorder accompanied by evidence-based treatment over the past several decades, the moral paradigm persists. Nurses can help disseminate this neurobiological information to patients about the neurobiological base for alcohol use disorders and treatments.

CLINICAL STRATEGIES FOR IDENTIFYING AND MANAGING ALCOHOL PROBLEMS

Nearly 3 decades have lapsed since Chick and colleagues[33(p697)] stated that, "screening for alcohol problems should become a routine part of nursing assessment and the medical history so that advice can be given before irreversible physical or psychosocial problems have developed." Despite recommendations and mandates, uptake of screening and brief intervention by health care providers in any health care setting is still relatively limited.[34] It is paramount that nurses be equipped with an understanding of a set of clinical strategies, known as screening, brief intervention, and referral to treatment (SBIRT).

To begin, it is important to acknowledge that the spectrum of problematic alcohol consumption ranges from risky alcohol use to alcohol use disorders (alcohol abuse and dependence). According to the National Institute on Alcohol Abuse and Alcoholism (NIAAA), maximum drinking limits for healthy men up to age 65 are no more than 4 standard drinks in a day *and* no more than 14 standard drinks in a week. The maximum limits for healthy women and healthy men over age 65 are no more than 3 standard drinks in a day *and* no more than 7 standard drinks in a week.[35] A general overview of SBIRT is provided herein. Several resources are available for nurses to obtain more detailed information and guidance related to SBIRT (**Box 1**).

Screening

The initial screening is important to determine if the number of standard drinks exceed the maximum limits (ie, 5 or more drinks in a day for men and 4 or more drinks in a day for women). Further screening, using a standardized, validated instrument, is indicated. The 10-item Alcohol Use Disorders Identification Test (AUDIT) and the 3-item AUDIT-C (AUDIT-Consumption) are the most extensively researched measures for accurately and practically screen for alcohol problems.[36] Although the original goal of the AUDIT was to identify hazardous drinking (ie, a level less severe than diagnosable alcohol abuse or dependence), evidence supports using the AUDIT to screen for alcohol dependence, with gender-specific cut points.[36] An AUDIT score $\geq$8 for men and $\geq$4 for women indicates a need to determine the weekly average of the number of days in which an alcoholic drink is consumed and the number of alcoholic drinks consumed on a typical day.[36]

Assessment

Informed by the screening results, the next step is to assess the severity and extent of alcohol-related symptoms. The NIAAA[35] clinical guide provides assessment questions

---

Box 1
Screening, brief interventions, and referral to treatment: resources for nurses

Addiction training for nurses: Screening, Brief Intervention, and Referral to Treatment (SBIRT)

- A continuing nursing education available at: http://www.nursing.pitt.edu/academics/ce/SBIRT.jsp (contact hours and fee).

Babor TF, Higgins-Biddle JC, Saunders JB, et al. The alcohol use disorders identification test: guidelines for use in primary care. Geneva (Switzerland): World Health Organization; 2001. Available at: www.who.org.

- Free manual with guidelines

Broyles LM, Gordon AJ, Kengor C, et al. A tailored curriculum of alcohol screening, brief intervention, and referral to treatment (SBIRT) for nurses in inpatient settings. J Addict Nurs, in press.

- Describes the *RN-SBIRT Training Curriculum*, a 2-h session followed by a single 30-min booster session

National Institute on Alcohol Abuse and Alcoholism. Helping patients who drink too much: a clinician's guide. National Institute on Alcohol Abuse and Alcoholism (NIAAA); 2005. Available at: http://pubs.niaaa.nih.gov/publications/Practitioner/CliniciansGuide2005/guide.pdf.

- Provides comprehensive guidance for nurses and other clinicians including clinician support and patient education materials, including the definition of a standard drink.
- A pocket guide for alcohol screening and brief intervention can be downloaded from http://pubs.niaaa.nih.gov/publications/Practitioner/PocketGuide/pocket.pdf.

Pating DR, Miller MM, Goplerud E, et al. New systems of care for substance use disorders. Psychiatr Clin North Am 2012;35:327–56.

- Provides a case study related to preventative care for the person with unhealthy alcohol use, along with a synopsis of screening and brief intervention.

that correspond with the criteria for alcohol abuse and alcohol dependence defined in the *Diagnostic and Statistical Manual of Mental Disorders*.[21] Affirmative response to one or more of the 4 items for alcohol abuse and 3 or more of the 7 items for alcohol dependence indicate the need for a brief intervention.

Brief Intervention

A brief intervention is a nonconfrontational, patient-centered approach that involves a 5- to 15-minute conversation to raise awareness of alcohol-related consequences and motivate a patient toward behavior change.[37] The brief intervention for alcohol abuse or dependence focuses on increasing patients' understanding of the severity and extent of their alcohol use and motivating behavior change. As standard nursing practice, the registered nurse collects comprehensive data pertinent to the health care consumer's health and/or the situation.[13] Thus, the nurse can address alcohol-related concerns within the context of the comprehensive physical, functional, psychosocial, and other areas of the assessment. The need for medically managed withdrawal and other alcohol specialty treatment should also be considered.

Referral to Treatment

Referral to treatment is recommended for patients who have alcohol use disorders or a history of alcohol treatment. In specialty treatment settings, patients access more extensive assessment and treatment.[37] In presenting a case for teaching patients about the neurobiological basis of addictions, Finnell[38] suggested that this information could be useful to empower patients, ease their defenses, and reduce the stigma they experience. Nevertheless, a wide gap remains between the advances in science related to the neurobiological base for alcohol use disorders and treatments and disseminating that information to patients.

DISSEMINATING NEUROBIOLOGICAL INFORMATION AS A BRIEF INTERVENTION

Information about the neurobiological base of alcohol disorders and their treatments can be woven into the conversation of a brief intervention as outlined in the NIAAA[35] clinician's guide. **Box 2** provides key points related to providing neurobiological information as a brief intervention.

OUTCOMES OF PROVIDING HEALTH INFORMATION

The importance of increasing patients' knowledge about their illness and treatment has been raised by others.[39,40] Recent decades have witnessed a growing emphasis on patients as active consumers of health information.[41] The Pew Internet and American Life Project[42] estimated that 113 million Americans have searched the Internet for health information. Traditionally, the patient had a passive role in making medical decisions with physicians playing the leading role.[43] However this approach has shifted to one whereby health care consumers are expected to take a more active role in reaching health care decisions, a switch that is possible due to an increase public access to an expanded range of medical information and sources.[44] Availability to access health information has empowered individuals as decision-makers who are evaluating the relative benefits and costs of preventive, diagnostic, and treatment options that are consistent with their preferences and values.[45] Likewise, patients with alcohol use disorders should have ready access to health information about the underpinnings of these chronic and relapsing disorders to help them recognize that they are not at fault, nor did they intend their alcohol consumption to reach such a point as to become an alcohol disorder.

Box 2
Conversation points in disseminating neurobiological information as a brief intervention

Address

- The reported consequences from the assessment
- The potential biologic, psychological, social, and spiritual consequences if not managed
- The point that consequences were not intended

Provide information to remove barriers to behavior change and barriers to treatment

- The roots/cause
  - The attraction to alcohol is brain-based
  - Chemicals interact with other chemicals. That is, alcohol as a chemical from the outside relates to chemicals on the inside through interactions within and between neurons of the brain. In turn, these chemical interactions affect feelings, thoughts, memories, and behaviors.
  - The attraction to alcohol, also known as craving, is the brain's attempt to create a balanced chemistry that has been out of balance.
  - Continuing to drink alcohol will make this imbalance worse and create more disturbance and dysfunction, physically, personally, and socially. The consequences will become more severe.
- The good news
  - This was neither your fault nor your intention. A chemical can only relate to another chemical.
  - The brain can heal in the absence of alcohol.
  - Treatment is about learning how to manage this disorder.
  - Treatment works.

Negotiate a goal:[a]

- "Would you be willing to consider making a change in your drinking?"[b]
- "Would you be willing to consider a referral to treatment?"
- "Would you be willing to consider a mutual help group?"
- "Would you be willing to consider a medication that is used to help people who want to abstain from alcohol?"[c]

Referral to treatment

- Locate referral resources in your area.[d] Become familiar with treatment providers and facilities providing evidence-based treatments, including pharmacotherapy. Inquire if they are disseminating information to patients about the neurobiological basis of alcohol disorders.
- Maintain access to a list of mutual help groups. Seek feedback from other patients about groups that are particularly supportive to their recovery.

Arrange follow-up

- Schedule appointment to review goals and maintain continuing support.

[a] Source for use of the readiness ruler: Coleman MT, Pasternak RH. Effective strategies for behavior change. Prim Care 2012;39:281–305.
[b] See NIAAA[35] (p. 7) regarding recommending abstaining or cutting down. Assess need for medically managed withdrawal and refer accordingly.
[c] See NIAAAA[35] (p. 13).
[d] See NIAAAA[35] (p. 23).

Within the context of the neurobiological evidence-based knowledge, nurses and other providers should approach their patients in a nonjudgmental manner, understanding the powerlessness that comes when the brain reward system is set in motion by alcohol consumption. This science-based approach to patients with alcohol disorders is important in promoting a positive patient-provider relationship. According to Falvo,[46] health professionals can build and promote a partnership with their patients through the communication and exchange of health information. Effective patient education occurs when there is mutual trust and respect, setting the stage for determining mutually agreed-on goals, identifying barriers that may stand in their way, and designing a plan of action.[46]

There is evidence that providing health information impacts health outcomes. For example, patients who never received diabetes education showed a striking increased risk of a major complication.[47] Nevertheless, complications associated with diabetes can be reduced when patients receive information on glucose monitoring, insulin injection technique, insulin storage, recognition/treatment of hypoglycemia, and how to manage their insulin injection and doses.[48] An Internet-based diabetes self-management program, designed to increase knowledge, provide skills, and enhance social support, found overall improvement, especially on dietary behaviors.[49] Grounded on providing health information, other programs that promote diabetes self-management encourage setting of personal goals and provide individualized feedback to assist patients in dealing with the challenges of self-care.[50–52]

The significance of providing health information to patients has also been stressed in other chronic diseases such as Hepatitis C (HCV). McKay and colleagues[53] noted that, following HCV education, patients' posttest scores improved by 14%, specifically in the areas of HCV transmission, general knowledge, and health care maintenance. Importantly with respect to ongoing surveillance and treatment, there were high rates of follow-through for liver specialty clinic attendance.[53] Other studies have found that providing HCV education resulted in a marked increase in willingness to accept HCV treatment.[54,55] These findings are encouraging for nurses providing information about the neurobiological base of alcohol use disorders with respect to increasing patients' awareness of the cause of the disorder and evidence-based treatments, with the goal of promoting acceptance of referral to treatment, engagement in, and follow-through with alcohol treatment.

Among patients with alcohol disorder, research is needed to evaluate the impact of providing the neurobiological information on their acceptance of referral to treatment, engagement in treatment, completion of treatment, short-term and long-term alcohol consumption, and on their sustained recovery.

SUMMARY

Alcohol use disorders are associated with a high human and economic cost. Although some will be able to decrease alcohol consumption, abstain from alcohol, and recover fully, specialty treatment will be necessary for most. The small proportion of those who get this life-saving treatment is concerning. Nurses have extended patient contact, are regular and stable providers in most health care settings, have a holistic focus of practice, have a solid grounding in health problems that are common comorbid conditions in individuals consuming any amount of alcohol, and are recognized as the most trusted profession. Nurses can integrate information about the neurobiological base of alcohol disorders in their conversations with these at-risk individuals. Through these conversations, nurses can be instrumental in reducing the barriers to the patient's acceptance of referral to specialty alcohol treatment.

REFERENCES

1. Centers for Disease Control and Prevention. Alcohol Related Disease Impact (ARDI) application. 2008. Available at: http://apps.nccd.cdc.gov/DACH_ARDI/Default.aspx. Accessed November 15, 2012.
2. Rehm J, Mathers C, Popova S, et al. Alcohol and global health 1: Global burden of disease and injury and economic cost attributable to alcohol use and alcohol-use disorders. Lancet 2009;373:2223–33.
3. Finnell DS. A clarion call for nurse-led SBIRT across the continuum of care. Alcohol Clin Exp Res 2012;36:1134–8.
4. Institute of Medicine (IOM). The future of nursing: leading change, advancing health. Washington, DC: The National Academies Press; 2011.
5. World Health Organization. Management of substance abuse: Alcohol. Available at: http://www.who.int/substance_abuse/facts/alcohol/en/index.html. Accessed November 15, 2012.
6. Bouchery EE, Harwood HJ, Sacks JJ, et al. Economic costs of excessive alcohol consumption in the US, 2006. Am J Prev Med 2011;41:516–24.
7. Office of Applied Studies. Results from the 2002 National Survey on Drug Use and Health: National findings (DHHS Publication No. SMA 03–3836, NSDUH Series H-22). Rockville (MD): Substance Abuse and Mental Health Services Administration; 2003.
8. Office of Applied Studies. Results from the 2003 National Survey on Drug Use and Health: National findings (DHHS Publication No. SMA 04–3964, NSDUH Series H-25). Rockville (MD): Substance Abuse and Mental Health Services Administration; 2004.
9. Office of Applied Studies. Results from the 2004 National Survey on Drug Use and Health: National findings (DHHS Publication No. SMA 05–4062, NSDUH Series H-28). Rockville (MD): Substance Abuse and Mental Health Services Administration; 2005.
10. Substance Abuse and Mental Health Services Administration, Office of Applied Studies. The NSDUH Report: alcohol treatment: need, utilization, and barriers 2009. Rockville (MD). Available at: http://www.oas.samhsa.gov/2k9/AlcTX/AlcTX.pdf. Accessed November 15, 2012.
11. Mojtabai R, Crum RM. Perceived unmet need for alcohol and drug use treatments and future use of services: results from a longitudinal study. Drug Alcohol Depend 2013;127(1–3):59–64.
12. Rubenstein LV, Chaney EF, Ober S, et al. Using evidence-based quality improvement methods for translating depression collaborative care research into practice. Fam Syst Health 2010;28:91–113.
13. American Nurses Association. Nursing: Scope and Standards of Practice. Silver Spring (MD): American Nurses Association; 2010.
14. Azevedo FA, Carvalho LR, Grinberg LT, et al. Equal numbers of neuronal and nonneuronal cells make the human brain an isometrically scaled-up primate brain. J Comp Neurol 2009;513:532–41.
15. Pakkenberg B, Pelvig D, Marner L, et al. Aging and the human neocortex. Exp Gerontol 2003;38:95–9.
16. Pierce RC, Kumaresan V. The mesolimbic dopamine system: The final common pathway for the reinforcing effect of drugs of abuse? Neurosci Biobehav Rev 2006;30:215–38.
17. Urban NB, Martinez D. Neurobiology of addiction: insight from neurochemical imaging. Psychiatr Clin North Am 2012;35:521–41.

18. Erickson CK. The science of addiction: from neurobiology to treatment. New York: W. W. Norton & Company Inc; 2007.

19. DeHaan HJ. Origins and import of reinforcing self-stimulation of the brain. J Hist Neurosci 2010;19:24–32.

20. Feduccia AA, Chatterjee S, Bartlett SE. Neuronal nicotinic acetylcholine receptors: neuroplastic changes underlying alcohol and nicotine addictions. Front Mol Neurosci 2012;5:83.

21. American Psychiatric Association. Diagnostic and statistical manual of mental disorders. Text Revision (DSM-IV-TR). 4th edition. Washington, DC: American Psychiatric Association; 2010.

22. Belin D. Addictions—from pathophysiology to treatment. Rijeka (Croatia); 2012.

23. Volkow ND, Baler RD, Goldstein RZ. Addiction: pulling at the neural threads of social behaviors. Neuron 2011;69:599–602.

24. Potenza MN, Sofuoglu M, Carroll KM. Neuroscience of behavioral and pharmacological treatments for addictions. Neuron 2011;69:696–712.

25. Leggio L. Understanding and treating alcohol craving and dependence: recent pharmacological and neuroendocrinological findings. Alcohol Alcohol 2009;44: 341–52.

26. Petrakis IL. A rational approach to the pharmacotherapy of alcohol dependence. J Clin Psychopharmacol 2006;26:S3–12.

27. Dutra L, Stathopoulou G, Basden SL, et al. A meta-analytic review of psychosocial interventions for substance use disorders. Am J Psychiatry 2008;165: 179–87.

28. Magill M, Ray LA. Cognitive-behavioral treatment with adult alcohol and illicit drug users: a meta-analysis of randomized controlled trials. J Stud Alcohol Drugs 2009;70(4):516–27.

29. Tolin DF. Is cognitive-behavioral therapy more effective than other therapies? A meta-analytic review. Clin Psychol Rev 2010;30(6):710–20.

30. Adinoff B, Iranmanesh A, Veldhuis J, et al. Disturbances of the stress response: the role of the HPA axis during alcohol withdrawal and abstinence. Alcohol Health Res World 1998;22:67–72.

31. Adinoff B, Ruether K, Krebaum S, et al. Increased salivary cortisol concentrations during chronic alcohol intoxication in a naturalistic clinical sample of men. Alcohol Clin Exp Res 2003;27:1420–7.

32. Clarke TK, Treutlein J, Zimmermann US, et al. HPA-axis activity in alcoholism: examples for a gene-environment interaction. Addict Biol 2008;13:1–14.

33. Chick J, Lloyd G, Crombie E. Counselling problem drinkers in medical wards: a controlled study. Br Med J (Clin Res Ed) 1985;290:965–7.

34. Kuehn BM. Despite benefit, physicians slow to offer brief advice on harmful alcohol use. JAMA 2008;299:751–3.

35. National Institute on Alcohol Abuse and Alcoholism. Helping patients who drink too much: a clinician's guide. National Institute on Alcohol Abuse and Alcoholism (NIAAA); 2005. Available at: http://pubs.niaaa.nih.gov/publications/Practitioner/CliniciansGuide2005/guide.pdf. Accessed November 15, 2012.

36. Reinert DF, Allen JP. The Alcohol Use Disorders Identification Test (AUDIT): an update of research findings. Alcohol Clin Exp Res 2007;31:185–99.

37. Sullivan E, Fleming M. TIP 24: a guide to substance abuse services for primary care clinicians. Rockville (MD): U.S. Department of Health and Human Services, Substance Abuse and Mental Health Services Administration; 1997. DHHS Publication No. (SMA). Available at: http://www.taadas.org/publications/prodimages/TIP%2024.pdf. Accessed November 15, 2012.

38. Finnell DS. The case for teaching patients about the neurobiological basis of addictions. J Addict Nurs 2000;12:149–58.
39. Buchanan DR. Perspective: a new ethic for health promotion: reflections on a philosophy of health education for the 21st century. Health Educ Behav 2006; 33:290–304.
40. Rummel-Kluge C, Pitschel-Walz G, Buml J, et al. Psychoeducation in schizophrenia: results of a survey of all psychiatric institutions in Germany, Austria, and Switzerland. Schizophr Bull 2006;32:765–75.
41. Arnetz JE, Winblad U, Arnetz BB, et al. Physicians' and nurses' perceptions of patient involvement in myocardial infarction care. Eur J Cardiovasc Nurs 2008;7: 113–20.
42. Fox S. Pew Internet and American life project. Online health search [webpage]. Available at: http://www.pewinternet.org/Reports/2006/Online-Health-2006. Accessed November 15, 2012.
43. Brody DS. The patient's role in clinical decision-making. Ann Intern Med 1980; 93:718–22.
44. Dutta-Bergman MJ. Access to the internet in the context of community participation and community satisfaction. New Media Soc 2005;7:89–109.
45. Kaplan RM, Frosch DL. Decision making in medicine and health care. Annu Rev Clin Psychol 2005;1:525–56.
46. Falvo DR. Effective patient education: a guide to increased compliance. 4th edition. Mississauga (Canada): Jones & Bartlett Publishers; 2010.
47. Nicolucci A, Cavaliere D, Scorpiglione N, et al. A comprehensive assessment of the avoidability of long-term complications of diabetes. Diabetes Care 1996;19: 927–33.
48. Inzucchi SE, Bergenstal RM, Buse JB, et al. Management of hyperglycaemia in type 2 diabetes: a patient-centered approach. Position statement of the American Diabetes Association (ADA) and the European Association for the Study of Diabetes (EASD). Diabetologia 2012;55:1577–96.
49. Mckay HG, King D, Eakin EG, et al. The diabetes network internet-based physical activity intervention: a randomized pilot study. Diabetes Care 2001;24: 1328–34.
50. Glasgow RE, Eakin EG. Medical office-based interventions. In: Snoek FJ, Skinner CS, editors. Psychological aspects of diabetes care. London: Wiley; 2000. p. 142–68.
51. Johnson JD. Cancer-related information seeking. Cresskill (NJ): Hampton Press; 1997.
52. Toobert DJ, Glasgow RE. Problem-solving and diabetes self-care. Int J Behav Med 1991;14:71–86.
53. McKay HG, Glasgow RE, Feil EG, et al. Internet-based diabetes self-management and support: initial outcomes from the Diabetes Network Project. Rehabil Psychol 2002;47:31–48.
54. Balfour L, Cooper C, Tasca GA, et al. Evaluation of health care needs and patient satisfaction among hepatitis C patients treated at a hospital-based, viral hepatitis clinic. Can J Public Health 2004;95:272–7.
55. Gupta K, Romney D, Briggs M, et al. Effects of a brief educational program on knowledge and willingness to accept treatment among patients with hepatitis C at inner-city hospitals. J Community Health 2007;32:221–30.

Understanding Alcoholism

Albert Rundio Jr, PhD, DNP, RN, APRN, CARN-AP, NEA-BC[a,b,c,*]

KEYWORDS

- Alcoholism • Ethyl alcohol • Methyl alcohol • Alcohol abuse

KEY POINTS

- Ethanol is an ingredient that is intoxicating in nature.
- Alcohol is rapidly absorbed from the stomach, small intestine, and colon.
- Abuse of alcohol affects nearly every body system.
- Primary care providers are critical to diagnosing alcoholism.

This article provides an introduction to the health effects of alcoholism. Discussed are ethyl alcohol and methyl alcohol.

The National Survey on Drug Use and Health found that about 18.7 million Americans were dependent on or abused alcohol in 2005.[1] The 2011 National Survey of Drug Use and Health for ages 12 and older demonstrated that 82.2% of children ages 12 or older drink alcohol. Sixty-six percent had used alcohol within the past year, and 51.8% had used alcohol within the past month.[2]

HISTORICAL DEVELOPMENT

Ethanol is an ingredient that is intoxicating in nature. This ingredient can be found in wine, liquor, and beer. The primary production of alcohol is through the fermentation of sugars, starches, and yeast. Alcohol is not considered an illicit drug when one is of legal age to drink. Alcohol is a central nervous depressant.[3]

Consumption of alcoholic beverages has a long history. Ten thousand years ago beer was made from grain. This process was discovered accidentally. In 1100 AD a guild was formed devoted to brewing beer. Eight thousand years ago, wine was consumed. Five thousand years ago vineyards were grown to make wine. In 2000 BC Hammurabi, the leader of Babylon, established rules for the sale and purchase of wine. In Ancient Greek culture, Dionysus/Bacchus was the god of wine. An alchemist in the sixteenth century discovered that alcohol was the essence from distillation (distilled spirits). During the middle of the eighteenth century alcohol assumed the current meaning of the intoxicating ingredient of many common beverages.[3]

[a] Drexel University, 1505 Race Street, Room #429, Philadelphia, PA 19102, USA; [b] International Nurses Society on Addictions, PO Box 14846, Lenexa, KS 66285-4846, USA; [c] Lighthouse at Mays Landing, 5034 Atlantic Avenue, Mays Landing, NJ 08330, USA
* Drexel University, 1505 Race Street, Room #429, Philadelphia, PA 19102.
E-mail address: aar27@drexel.edu

Nurs Clin N Am 48 (2013) 385–390
http://dx.doi.org/10.1016/j.cnur.2013.05.001
0029-6465/13/$ – see front matter © 2013 Elsevier Inc. All rights reserved.

To further demonstrate this ancient awareness of intoxicating beverages, one can refer to the Bible. In Judges 13:3–4 it is stated: "you will conceive and bear a son… now then be careful to take no wine or strong drink and to eat nothing unclean."[4]

According to the National Institute on Drug Abuse, alcohol is the number one drug of choice for American youth, yet the seriousness of alcoholism does not register with the general public or policymakers.[5]

PRODUCTION OF ALCOHOL

The process for making alcohol begins by fermenting sugar to alcohol and then carbon dioxide. A significant portion of the US population abuses alcohol because alcohol is not a controlled substance. In some states alcohol is available in grocery markets and gas stations. In other states alcohol is only available at a licensed liquor store. The age when one can begin drinking varies from state to state. For example, in New Jersey, one cannot consume alcohol legally until the age of 21. Some individuals have a problem with this because the legal definition of an adult occurs at the age of 18, and certainly 18 year olds fight in wars for our country, yet in some states cannot legally purchase alcohol. The statistics on the dollar amount spent on the purchase of wine, beer, and liquor and advertisements for these products in the United States is staggering.

ABSORPTION

Alcohol is rapidly absorbed from the stomach, small intestine, and colon. The maximal blood concentration is achieved within 30 to 90 minutes of ingestion. Alcohol can also be absorbed through the lungs. Alcohol is uniformly distributed throughout tissues and body fluids. Alcohol readily crosses the placenta with exposure to the fetus. Alcohol is primarily eliminated through the renal system, the urinary tract, exhalation, and metabolism. When alcohol is consumed, it passes from the stomach and intestines into the blood; this process is referred to as absorption. Alcohol is then metabolized by enzymes, which are body chemicals that break down and speed-up the reaction of other chemicals. The liver is the primary target organ that breaks down alcohol consumption. In the liver, an enzyme known as alcohol dehydrogenase mediates the conversion of alcohol to acetylaldehyde. This is then rapidly converted to acetate by other enzymes and is eventually metabolized to carbon dioxide and water. Alcohol is also metabolized in the liver by the enzyme cytochrome P450IIE1 (CYP2E1) system, which may be increased after chronic drinking. Most alcohol that is consumed is metabolized in the liver, but the small quantity that remains unmetabolized permits alcohol concentration to be measured in the breath and the urine. The liver can metabolize only a certain amount of alcohol per hour regardless of the amount that is being consumed. The rate of alcohol metabolism depends in part on the amount of metabolizing enzymes in the liver, which varies among individuals. There seems to be genetic determinants. In general, after the consumption of one standard drink the amount of alcohol in the drinker's blood, which is referred to as the blood alcohol concentration, peaks within 30 to 45 minutes after ingestion. A standard drink is defined as 12 oz of beer; 8 oz of malt liquor; 5 oz of wine; or 1.5 oz of 80-proof of distilled spirits (a shot of liquor), all of which contain relatively the same amount of alcohol.[5]

The enzyme responsible for converting ethanol to acetylaldehyde is known as alcohol dehydrogenase. Acetaldehyde dehydrogenase (ALDH) is the enzyme for converting acetylaldehyde to acetate. There are genetic variations in ALDH, and variations among whites, African Americans, and Asians. Fifty percent of Asians have inactive

ALDH. Thus, 50% of this population has elevated acetylaldehyde levels after consumption of alcohol. The results of this are increased flushing, tachycardia, nausea and vomiting, and hyperventilation. The Asian population thus tends to have lower incidences of alcoholism secondary to this untoward unpleasant affect of alcohol consumption. One of the relapse prevention medications known as disulfiram (Antabuse) inhibits ALDH, thus causing the same type of unpleasant reaction that the Asian population experiences. Eighty percent to 90% of the alcohol is metabolized. The rate generally remains constant. The rate does not increase secondary to increased concentrations of alcohol in the blood. In general, about 30 mL equivalent to 1 oz is metabolized about every 3 hours. Females tend to have higher blood alcohol levels compared with males. Males tend to have higher stomach metabolism of alcohol compared with females.

ALCOHOL DEPENDENCE

Alcohol dependence is characterized by the following:

- Craving: A strong need for compulsion to drink; loss of control; the inability to limit one's drinking on any given occasion
- Tolerance: The need to drink greater and greater amounts of alcohol to get the same "high." Approximately 18,000,000 Americans meet the diagnostic criteria for alcohol abuse or alcoholism.[1]
- Physical dependence: This includes withdrawal symptoms, such as nausea, diaphoresis, shakiness, and anxiety. This occurs when alcohol is abruptly stopped after a period of heavy drinking.

Alcohol withdrawal effects include the following: tremor, nausea, irritability, agitation, hypertension, tachycardia, hallucinations, periods of blackout, and seizures. Some patients also experience a mildly elevated temperature.

EFFECTS OF ALCOHOLISM

Abuse of alcohol affects nearly every bodily system, including gastrointestinal system, cardiovascular system, metabolic system, central nervous system, hematopoietic system, and nutritional deficiencies. The common effects on the gastrointestinal system include esophagitis, gastritis, peptic ulcer, diarrhea, and pancreatitis. Because alcohol is metabolized in the liver the effects on the liver include fatty degeneration, alcoholic hepatitis, and eventual cirrhosis. Cirrhosis of the liver results from chronic abuse of alcohol. Ninety percent of cases of cirrhosis are attributable to alcohol. It is one of leading causes of death in the United States. The amount and duration of alcohol ingestion required to cause cirrhosis varies among individuals and between males and females. Ingestion of more than one pint of 80 proof alcohol daily for 10 years is associated with a 10% risk of cirrhosis and up to 50% after 25 years of the same pattern of use. Esophageal varices result secondary to portal hypertension, which may become irreversible and variceal bleeding is often the immediate cause of death. Patients with cirrhosis may also experience hypoglycemia and acidosis. Hypoglycemia results from limited glycogen storage in the high reduced nicotinamide/adenine dinucleotide ratio that depresses gluconeogenesis. Acidosis results from increased free fatty acid use, the synthesis of ketone bodies, and exaggerated lactic acid production with exercise. There also is a noted decreased absorption of essential vitamins, such as vitamin B_1, folate, vitamin B_{12}, and calcium. Cardiovascular system effects include exacerbation of angina and heart failure, hypertension, cardiomyopathies, and cardiac dysrhythmias. One of the common causes of cardiac dysrhythmias is decreased magnesium levels. Metabolic changes include ketoacidosis, lactic acidosis, hypomagnesemia, hypocalcemia, hypokalemia, hyperuricemia, and hypertriglyceridemia. Central nervous system changes include the following: acute intoxication, amnesia, cerebellar degeneration, Marchiafava-Bignami disease, central pontine myelinosis, cerebral atrophy, and myopathy. Withdrawal syndromes include tremulousness, hallucinations, seizures, and delirium tremens. Nutritional deficiencies include Wernicke-Korsakoff syndrome, folate deficiency, and pellagra. Vitamin B_1 deficiency is the causative factors of Wernicke encephalopathy. This illness is characterized by ocular disturbances, ataxia, and confusion. This illness has a 10% to 20% mortality rate. Korsakoff psychoses are characterized by cognitive dysfunction, loss of recent memory, the inability to learn new information, and are thought to be a chronic form of Wernicke encephalopathy. Hematopoietic system changes include anemia (a direct toxic effect of alcohol, folate deficiency, or iron deficiency anemia from chronic gastrointestinal bleeding) and thrombocytopenia. Alcohol consumption increases the risk of cancer, particularly in the oral cavity, pharynx and larynx, esophagus, and the liver. Subtle problems with alcoholism include lost productivity, impaired performance, motor impairment, and the increased cost to society in general. Nutritional deficiencies, in particular thiamine and vitamin B_{12}, occur despite good dietary intake. These deficiencies result from the direct toxicity of alcohol, impaired absorption and use of nutrients, and toxicity of alcohol metabolites with resulting neuropathies, bone marrow toxicity, cognitive changes, and intracranial hemorrhages. In the malnourished alcoholic, the resumption of a regular diet can cause severe rhabdomyolysis, hemolysis, and cellular hypoxia secondary to acute hypophosphatemia associated with the cellular uptake of glucose. The underlying thiamine vitamin B_1 deficiency is accentuated with the cellular uptake of glucose. Electrolyte disturbances including potassium, magnesium, and phosphate deficiencies are common in nutritionally compromised alcoholics. Other complications of alcoholism include social and psychological domains, such as family discord, poor employment history, legal difficulties, physical trauma, mood disorders, serious metabolic disturbances, and pathologic effects on the diversity of organs as previously described.

DIAGNOSING ALCOHOLISM

Primary care providers are critical to diagnosing alcoholism. Primary care providers need to be tuned to and assess patients for substance use disorders inclusive of alcoholism. They need to evaluate where the patient's use occurs and the method of use. They need to assess patients for prior treatment, family issues, and if the patient has a history of depression or suicide ideation. Patients with legal issues or financial issues may have a problem with alcoholism. Primary care providers should be tuned to job issues (eg, multiple excused absences could indicate a problem with alcoholism). Primary care providers need to be tuned to intoxication-related injuries, such as automobile accidents. They need to be tuned to patients who have a history of driving under the influence. They need to be tuned to patients with gastrointestinal symptoms, such as gastritis, which could be alcohol induced. They need to pay attention to laboratory values because elevated liver function studies can be a sign of alcoholism. They also need to be tuned to patients who have blackout periods and excessive requests for excuse notes from work or school. Primary care providers need to be tuned to insomnia that could be secondary to alcohol abuse. They need to be tuned to the patient's early morning tremors, depressive symptoms or lability of mood, or remorse related to alcohol and drug episodes. Primary care providers need to be tuned to alcohol on a patient's breath, or significant others complaining about the patient's drinking or drugging habits, and deterioration in work or school performance. A simple tool called the CAGE questionnaire can be used. The "C" in this tool stands for: Have you tried to "cut down" on your drinking? The "A" stands for: Are you "annoyed" by people telling you to stop drinking? The "G" stands for: Do you feel "guilty" about your drinking? The "E" stands for an "eye-opener": Do you drink on first getting up in the morning? Any two or more yes responses indicate a positive test, and that the patient could benefit from treatment. Treatment facilities generally use a CIWA scale (institute withdrawal scale for assessment of alcohol). This is an objective scale that provides a numeric score to determine in what stage of withdrawal is the alcoholic. The scores in this tool can be used to guide treatment with pharmacologic agents for detoxification.

FETAL ALCOHOL SYNDROME

Fetal alcohol syndrome (FAS) is one of the most preventable causes of adverse central nervous system development. A fair amount of infants are affected by FAS each year. Use of alcohol or illicit drugs during pregnancy has been linked to adverse birth outcomes, such as low birth weight, preterm delivery, and FAS.[6]

The National Institute on Alcohol Abuse and Alcoholism states that the prevalence of alcohol-related birth defects and alcohol-related neurobehavioral disorders (ARND) is expected to be significantly greater than the prevalence of FAS. Data recently analyzed by a National Institute on Alcohol Abuse and Alcoholism supported study on pregnancy and alcohol estimated that there was a threefold higher incidence of ARND than FAS. The study estimated that there are 9 cases per 1000 births of ARND, whereas FAS cases are estimated to be 0.6 to 3 cases per 1000 births.[6]

The characteristics of FAS include the following: growth retardation, craniofacial malformations, infants with a small head, and markedly reduced intelligence. FAS effects about 1 to every 3 births per 1000 births worldwide. In 1968, French researchers at the University of Nantes were the first to describe FAS. In the early 1970s, FAS was recognized as a condition at the University of Washington. A milder form of FAS also affects several infants per year in the United States. In this milder form of FAS, the characteristics include growth deficiency, learning dysfunction, and nervous system disabilities. Prenatal alcohol ingestion can have marked effects on the neonatal brain. The classic features of FAS include the following: a small head, underdeveloped pinna, a short nose, small eye openings, missing groove above the upper lip, a flat face, pointed small chin, and thin lips. Research in laboratories using mouse models also clearly demonstrates the difference between a normal mouse head and a mouse that has FAS.

ALCOHOL AND CANCER

Alcohol increases the risk of certain types of cancer. The primary systems that are affected include the oral cavity, the larynx and the pharynx, the esophagus, and the liver.

TREATMENT

Patients who abuse alcohol on a daily or almost daily basis benefit most from inpatient treatment at an addiction treatment center. Therapy is centered on a safe, medically monitored detoxification that is done over a period of time (usually 5–7 days). Use of benzodiazepines is the hallmark of detoxification. Patients also require psychological treatment and therapy. Group milieu therapy is used. Individual and group counseling and education sessions are used. Families also attend family programs. Many programs use the 12-step philosophy. After in-patient treatment, patients are dispositioned accordingly. Many are referred to intensive outpatient programs; some may be referred to long-term rehabilitation facilities and others are referred to half-way houses.

The goal of treatment is the maintenance of long-term sobriety. Alcoholism is a chronic disease, and, as such, some patients do relapse. Early entry back to treatment is most beneficial in these patients.

REFERENCES

1. Substance Abuse and Mental Health Services Administration, Office of Applied Studies. Results from the 2005 National Survey on Drug Use and Health: national findings 2006 (NSDUH Series H-30, DHHS Publication No. SMA 06-4194). Rockville (MD), Table G.29. Available at: http://www.samhsa.gov. Accessed April 24, 2013.
2. 2011 National Survey of Drug Use and Health (NSDUH) for Ages 12 and Older. Available at: http://www.drugabuse.gov/drugs-abuse/alcohol. Accessed April 24, 2013.
3. Gilbert SG. A small dose of alcohol. 2004. Available at: http://toxipedia.org/display/dose/Alcohol. Accessed April 26, 2013.
4. The Holy Bible. Judges: 13:3–4. In: Gilbert SG, editor. A small dose of alcohol. Available at: http://toxipedia.org/display/dose/Alcohol. Accessed April 26, 2013.
5. National Institute on Drug Abuse. Available at: http://www.nida.gov. Accessed April 24, 2013.
6. National Institute of Alcohol Abuse and Alcoholism (NIAAA) ICCFASD 1996-2000 Annual Report and 2001-2005 Strategic Plan. Available at: www.niaaa.nih.gov. Accessed April 24, 2013.

Implementing an Evidence-Based Detoxification Protocol for Alcoholism in a Residential Addictions Treatment Facility

Albert Rundio Jr, PhD, DNP, RN, APRN, CARN-AP, NEA-BC[a,b,c,*]

KEYWORDS

- Nurse executive • Nurse practitioner • Advanced practice nurse
- Chemical dependency • Substance abuse • Detoxification • Detoxification protocol
- Illicit drugs

KEY POINTS

- Addiction fits a Biopsychosocial/Spritual Disease Model.
- One of the primary goals of treatment is to address the components of this model.
- Benzodiazepines are the preferred pharmacologic agents for the treatment of acute alcohol withdrawal states.
- Relapse prevention incorporates the use of other types of pharmacologic agents.

INTRODUCTION/BACKGROUND OF ADDICTIONS

Substance use and abuse is not a new phenomenon in the US population. For years, Americans have used and abused various substances. Certain substances that are illegal today were not once always that way. For example, it is well known that Coca-Cola was a healing tonic that initially contained cocaine because small amounts of cocaine would give one more energy and stamina. Today, cocaine is termed an illicit or illegal substance, yet it is one of the most abused substances in our society. According to survey data from the National Household Survey on Drug Abuse,[1] 16.6 million persons age 12 years and older were classified with dependency on or abuse of alcohol or illicit drugs, which translates to approximately 7.3% of the population. Alcohol is considered a legal substance if one is of age. The age whereby alcohol becomes legal can vary by state laws. The economic impact of substance abuse was

[a] College of Nursing & Health Professions, Drexel University, 1505 Race Street, Room #429, Philadelphia, PA 19102, USA; [b] International Nurses Society on Addictions, PO Box 14846, Lenexa, KS 66285-4846, USA; [c] Lighthouse at Mays Landing, 5034 Atlantic Avenue, Mays Landing, NJ 08330, USA
* College of Nursing & Health Professions, Drexel University, 1505 Race Street, Room #429, Philadelphia, PA 19102.
E-mail address: aar27@drexel.edu

Nurs Clin N Am 48 (2013) 391–400
http://dx.doi.org/10.1016/j.cnur.2013.04.001
0029-6465/13/$ – see front matter © 2013 Elsevier Inc. All rights reserved.

estimated to have increased by 5.9% between 1992 and 1998 with the reported financial impact of substance abuse costing approximately 143.4 billion dollars in 1998.[2]

Alcoholism affects nearly 10% of the population in the United States and in European countries[3] (Hupkens and colleagues[4]). According to Phillips and coworkers,[5] nearly 1 in 10 adults (9.6%) or 8.2 million Americans excessively consume alcohol; men who are between the ages of 18 to 21 triple the incidence rate to 26%. Fifteen percent to 20% of all primary care and hospitalized patients are dependent on alcohol; one-fifth of the total national expenditure for hospital care is secondary to alcohol dependency, and approximately 50% of trauma patients have a history of alcohol dependency. Young adult men comprise the largest group of traumatized alcohol-dependent patients; a comorbid history of alcoholism is associated more frequently with trauma-related death than any other disease process, and alcohol-dependent patients frequently have prolonged intensive care unit admissions characterized by major complications.

Many attempts have been made to control substance use in our nation. The first attempt was the Harrison Tax Act in 1914.[6] The most profound efforts were during the Nixon Administration in 1970 when the Uniform Controlled Substances Act was enacted.[6] This act mandated that drugs had to be categorized by Schedule I through V. Drugs in Schedule I were illegal and had no medicinal use, for example, heroin. Drugs in Schedule V were safe for use. Under this act, the Drug Enforcement Administration was created in 1973 to monitor compliance with the act.[7] Practitioners, such as physicians, were now mandated to get Drug Enforcement Administration numbers for the prescribing of controlled substances. This, of course, has now expanded to include advanced practice nurses (APNs) such as nurse practitioners, who have prescribing rights for controlled dangerous substances. This act has focused primarily on law enforcement to control dangerous substances and those providers who violate prescription privileges.

Attempts have also been made to control alcoholism. Most legislation addresses DUIs (driving while intoxicated) and controlling the age that one can begin drinking. For example, New Jersey has some of the most stringent alcohol laws. One can not legally drink until the age of 21. Severe punishment results for DUIs inclusive of jail time and the loss of a driver's license for a 10-year time period for a third DUI offense. Nevertheless, with all of our efforts, substance use and abuse continues to be a major problem confronting US society.

A MODEL FOR ADDICTION

Addiction fits a Biopsychosocial/Spriitual Disease Model. Current research in the field has reinforced the biologic components to this disease process. For several years now, health practitioners have been aware that addiction is a "real" disease. Addicts do not elect to become addicted. With the advent of positive emission tomography scanning and functional magnetic resonance imaging, brain chemistry and neuro-chemical transmitter release have been studied. Many receptor sites in the primitive brain area called the ventral trigeminal area have been identified, for example, opium receptors, cocaine receptors, and alcohol receptors. Some theories on addiction are that clients may have damaged receptor sites or genetic mutations that affect neuro-chemical release and saturation of receptor sites. Certainly the psychology of the individual as well as the sociologic manifestations also contributes to addiction. Spirituality has brought many individuals to recovery. It is one of the founding philosophies of 12-step programs. Experiential data have demonstrated that many clients do not relate to any spiritual entity when they are addicted.

The best way to view addictions is to view it as a chronic disease process. This model certainly fits addictions. Just as a diabetic may have a high blood sugar after ingesting a large piece of cake, addicts also can relapse and turn back to substance use and abuse. Providers need to be understanding of patients who relapse because any chronic disorder can have reoccurrences. Clinicians should not judge individuals who relapse, but rather support their recovery until it is permanent.

One of the primary goals of treatment is to address the components of this model. The biologic aspect of addictions is accomplished through pharmacology for both detoxification and relapse prevention. The psychological component is addressed through psychiatric evaluation of the client because many clients have an underlying psychiatric disorder. The social component is addressed by including the family and significant others in the treatment process. The goal of treatment is to get clients to lead a meaningful life that is inclusive of returning to work or finding employment. As with any disease process, family inclusiveness is necessary as family members can be enablers, which is contradictory to the philosophy of treatment. The spiritual component is addressed through 12-step meetings, such as Alcoholics Anonymous, where having a belief in a "higher power" is one of the founding principles in this process.

RATIONALE FOR DEVELOPMENT OF AN EVIDENCE-BASED PROTOCOL

The idea for the development of an evidence-based protocol for detoxification and relapse prevention of alcoholism resulted from one APN's practice in a residential treatment center in southern New Jersey. Before the development of this protocol, when a member of the medical staff was making rounds, they would have to write detoxification orders on a daily basis. It is essential that medications used for the purpose of detoxification of clients be weaned down gradually. Stopping such medication abruptly could result in the patient experiencing acute withdrawal symptoms. After years of practice, this APN recognized that most detoxification orders followed the same pattern on a daily basis. The APN and Director of Nursing at the facility explored the possibility of developing a detoxification protocol that would address the entire length of stay medical and nursing orders for a client admitted to the treatment facility. The Director of Nursing and the APN met with the Medical Director to see if he would agree to the development and clinical trial of such a protocol.

Garnering his support was vital to the continuation of this process. The Medical Director was in full agreement. The benefits to the development of such a protocol were inclusive of the following:

1. Standardized written order form that was computer generated
2. Standardized patient care protocol
3. Pharmacologic and other interventions based on current evidence in the field
4. Decrease in variation of both written orders and patient care
5. Measurement and evaluation of treatment interventions
6. Decrease in the time needed to write daily orders
7. Flexibility for change as new evidence is discovered.

A review of the literature was conducted so that an evidence-based protocol could be developed that addressed not only detoxification of the patient but also relapse prevention strategies.

REVIEW OF THE LITERATURE

According to Lejoyeux and colleagues,[8] benzodiazepines (BZDs) are the preferred pharmacologic agents for the treatment of acute alcohol withdrawal states. The authors further state that mild to moderate withdrawal symptoms can be treated with BZDs on an outpatient basis, whereas severe withdrawal states require inpatient admission. Lejoyeux and coworkers[8] state that BZDs do not improve abstinence rates and in most circumstances are not indicated for long-term use. A variety of BZDs can be used for successful detoxification. Librium is the gold standard for treatment of alcohol-withdrawal states. Ativan has also been used with success and is oftentimes the preferred treatment in the acute care hospital setting because Ativan can be administered intravenously. One of the problems with use of the BZDs is their long half-life. In some cases of patients with liver failure secondary to cirrhosis and alcoholism, BZDs given orally are not processed quickly enough by the failing liver. Serax as an alternative to BZD has been found to be more effective in these cases.

Phillips and colleagues[5] designed a process improvement project that developed an alcohol withdrawal syndrome (AWS) management protocol for the acute care hospital setting. The design of this project included a work team that comprised physicians, pharmacists, and nurses led by a behavioral health clinical nurse specialist. The outcome of this project was the development and integration of a safe and effective treatment protocol that effectively managed AWS. This project was facilitated by collaborative, evidence-based decision-making. The authors addressed the 3 following key components of care: (1) the identification of high-risk patients; (2) the initiation of prophylactic treatment; and (3) the initiation of effective and timely pharmacologic interventions in an effort to prevent medical complications in AWS that could lead to death. The authors also concluded from their review that BZDs are the mainstay of primary pharmacologic therapy in patients in AWS. Their preferred medication in the acute care setting was Diazepam.

Nimmerrichter and coworkers[9] conducted a double-blind controlled trail of γ–hydroxybutyrate (GHB) and Clomethiazole in the treatment of alcohol withdrawal symptoms. The purpose of the study was to assess GHB's efficacy and safety in ameliorating symptoms of alcohol withdrawal. Subjects were randomized to receive either Clomethizole or GHB. One Clomethizole group was established. Two GHB groups were formed whereby the dosage of the GHB varied by group. The authors concluded that there was no difference between the 3 treatment groups in the rating of alcohol withdrawal symptoms. There were also no requests for additional medication. After tapering of medication, there was no increase in withdrawal symptoms noted nor requests for medication, which was indicative that physical tolerance did not develop in any of the groups. The most frequently reported side effect was in the GHB group, which reported transient vertigo after the evening double dosage of medication. GHB used to be sold as a "health tonic" in health food stores until the potential for abuse was discovered. GHB overdose can cause cessation of respiration, coma, and death. GHB was pulled off of the market a few years ago. As a result of this, GHB is usually not found in treatment protocols for alcohol dependency.

Relapse prevention incorporates the use of other types of pharmacologic agents. Antabuse has been on the market for several years now. Many clinicians have stopped prescribing this medication secondary to life-threatening reactions inclusive of death in patients who drink alcohol when taking Antabuse. Streeton and Whelan[10] conducted a meta-analysis of Naltrexone use as a relapse prevention medication for alcoholism. The authors searched MEDLINE, EMBASE, PsychLIT, and Cochrane Controlled Trials Registry for articles published from 1976 to 2001. Their meta-analysis demonstrated that Naltrexone was superior to placebo. Subjects in the Naltrexone treatment groups maintained abstinence longer and had fewer episodes of relapse compared with those subjects in the control groups. In 2006, a pharmaceutical firm developed Vivitrol, an injectable form of Naltrexone. Vivitrol is administered on a once-monthly basis and is ideal for patients who have elevated liver enzymes because oral Naltrexone is contraindicated in such patients. Vivitrol must be ordered through the pharmaceutical firm that developed the medication and not at a standard retail pharmacy. Campral (Acamprosate) has also been demonstrated to be an effective relapse prevention medication for alcoholism. Although the exact mechanism of action is not completely understood, according to Ott and colleagues,[11] the available evidence suggests that it enhances the function of NMDA, an amino acid receptor. This medication is currently used in treatment as a relapse prevention medication because it improves abstinence outcome and diminishes cravings for alcohol. The standard dose of Campral is 666 mg 3 times daily administered orally.

Brown,[12] Liebson and colleagues,[13] and El-Bassel and colleagues[14] estimate that alcohol dependency rates vary from 5% to 49% among participants in Methadone Maintenance Programs. Caputo and colleagues[15] evaluated alcohol use in nonalcoholic heroin addicts during the first 4 weeks of a treatment program. The treatment program consisted of either a Methadone Maintenance Program or a Non-Methadone Maintenance Program. The authors note that many heroin-dependent clients will begin to abuse alcohol when in treatment. Three hundred fifty-nine heroin-addicted subjects were enrolled on an outpatient basis. All patients met the DSM-IV criteria. Thirty-two subjects dropped out of the study. The authors noted a significant decrease in the daily alcohol intake in the Methadone Maintenance Program compared to the Non-Methadone Maintenance Program. The authors concluded that the results of the study suggested a possible effect in reducing alcohol consumption by administering Methadone on a short-term basis to nonalcoholic heroin-addicted patients.

From review of the literature, it is apparent that BZDs are the mainstay for acute detoxification and Naltrexone, Campral, and Vivitrol are the primary medications that focus on relapse prevention along with psychotherapy and counseling.

IMPLEMENTATION OF AN EVIDENCE-BASED DETOXIFICATION PROTOCOL

Based on the evidence, the Director of Nursing had the APN develop a detoxification protocol for alcohol dependency. This protocol was reviewed by the Medical Director. The protocol was then implemented and evaluated for a 3-month time period. Patient outcomes were monitored (Appendix A). Medical staff and nursing staff satisfaction with the protocol were also monitored. The protocol was so successful that 2 additional alcohol protocols were developed for implementation with the goal of protocol development for all forms of substances (Appendices B–D).

This evidence-based practice has now become standard at this facility thanks to the foresight of a Director of Nursing and an APN, who recognized the value in treating patients based on current evidence.

APPENDIX A

Outcome Evaluation

Outcome evaluation will consist of direct observation and qualitative evaluation with use of a focus group of nurses.

I. Outcome Evaluation
   Quantitative & Qualitative Evaluation with Defined Indicators 3 months after implementation of project
   1. Direct observation of patients by nursing and medical staffs

2. Concurrent Chart Audit with Defined Indicators
   a. # of seizures
   b. Vital signs
   c. # of time P.R.N medications are used based on Clinical Institute Withdrawal Assessment of Alcohol Scale (CIWA)
   d. Pain Assessment Scale
   e. # of time detoxification protocols have to be readjusted
3. Qualitative Focus Group of Nursing Staff with Open-Ended Interview Questions

APPENDIX B

ADULT ALCOHOL DETOXIFICATION PROTOCOL # 1

Patient Name: _____ *ID#:* _____

1. Admit to:
2. Regular Diet
3. Vital signs per policy
4. Administer 0.1 cubic centimeters intradermally to left forearm Tuberculin Purified Protein Derivative; repeat in two weeks when applicable.
5. Multivitamins one tab orally daily for length of stay
6. Thiamine 100 milligrams orally twice daily for 5 Days, then
7. Thiamine 100 milligrams orally once daily thereafter for length of stay
8. Librium 75 milligrams orally as initial dose then
9. Librium 50 milligrams orally every 6 hours for 24 hours, then
10. Librium 35 milligrams orally every 6 hours for 24 hours, then
11. Librium 25 milligrams orally every 6 hours for 24 hours, then
12. Librium 10 milligrams orally every 6 hours for 24 hours, then discontinue
13. Librium 25 milligrams orally every 4 hours as needed based on signs and symptoms of withdrawal for 5 days
14. Levsin 0.125 milligrams sublingually every 6 hours as needed for abdominal cramps for 5 days
15. Vistaril 50 milligrams orally every 4 hours as needed for anxiety or agitation for length of stay
16. 48 hours after discontinuation of the detoxification protocol Campral 333 milligrams, (2 tablets) will be initiated orally three times per day
17. Trazodone 50 milligrams orally at bed time as needed for insomnia for length of stay
18. May repeat Trazodone 50 milligrams orally 1 additional dose 2 hours after the first dose if the first dose is not effective as needed for insomnia for length of stay
19. Milk of Magnesia 30 cubic centimeters orally twice daily as needed for constipation for length of stay
20. Maalox 30 cubic centimeters orally twice daily as needed for indigestion for length of stay
21. Kaopectate 30 cubic centimeters orally twice daily as needed for diarrhea for length of stay
22. Tylenol ii tabs orally three times daily as needed for headache and/or temp above 101° F for length of stay
23. Motrin 600 mg orally every 6 hours as needed for muscle aches and pain for length of stay

24. Robitussin 10 ml orally every 4 hours as needed for cough for length of stay
25. Cepacol throat lozenges one orally every 4 hours as needed for sore throat for length of stay
26. Random Urine Drug Screen (as determined by nursing)
27. Complete the CIWA (for alcohol) if considering administration of PRN detox medication.

Routine Labs: ____ CBC   ____Urinalysis
               ____ SMAC   ____Urine Drug Screen
               ____ Urine Pregnancy Test   ____Serum Pregnancy Test

Physician/APN Signature: _____ Date: _____ Time: _____.

NOTE: This protocol may be adjusted at any time by the Medical Staff.

APPENDIX C

ALCOHOL DETOXIFICATION PROTOCOL # 2

Patient Name: _____ *ID#:* _____

28. Admit to:
29. Regular Diet
30. Vital signs per policy
31. Administer 0.1 cubic centimeters intradermally to left forearm Tuberculin Purified Protein Derivative; repeat in two weeks when applicable.
32. Multivitamins one tab orally daily for length of stay
33. Thiamine 100 milligrams orally twice daily for 5 Days, then
34. Thiamine 100 milligrams orally once daily thereafter for length of stay
35. Librium 75 milligrams orally as initial dose then
36. Librium 75 milligrams orally every 6 hours for 24 hours, then
37. Librium 50 milligrams orally every 6 hours for 24 hours, then
38. Librium 35 milligrams orally every 6 hours for 24 hours, then
39. Librium 25 milligrams orally every 6 hours for 24 hours, then
40. Librium 10 milligrams orally every 6 hours for 24 hours, then discontinue
41. Librium 25 milligrams orally every 4 hours as needed based on signs and symptoms of withdrawal for 5 days, then discontinue
42. Levsin 0.125 milligrams sublingually every 6 hours as needed for abdominal pain for 5 days
43. Vistaril 50 milligrams orally every 4 hours as needed for anxiety or agitation for length of stay
44. 48 hours after discontinuation of the detoxification protocol Campral 333 milligrams, (2 tablets) will be initiated orally three times per day
45. Trazodone 50 milligrams orally at bed time as needed for insomnia for length of stay
46. May repeat Trazodone 50 milligrams orally 1 additional dose 2 hours after the first dose if the first dose is not effective as needed for insomnia for length of stay
47. Milk of Magnesia 30 cubic centimeters orally twice daily as needed for constipation for length of stay

48. Maalox 30 cubic centimeters orally twice daily as needed for indigestion for length of stay
49. Kaopectate 30 cubic centimeters orally twice daily as needed for diarrhea for length of stay
50. Tylenol ii tabs orally three times a day as needed for headache or temp above 101° F for length of stay
51. Motrin 600 milligrams orally every 6 hours as needed for muscle aches or pain for length of stay
52. Robitussin 10 milliliters orally every 4 hours as needed for cough for length of stay
53. Cepacol throat lozenges one orally every 4 hours as needed for sore throat for length of stay
54. Random Urine Drug Screen (as determined by nursing)
55. Complete the CIWA (for alcohol) if considering administration of PRN detox medication

NOTE: This protocol may be adjusted at any time by the Medical Staff.

Routine Labs: ____ CBC   ____Urinalysis
              ____ SMAC   ____Urine Drug Screen
              ____ Urine Pregnancy Test   ____Serum Pregnancy Test

Physician/APN Signature: _____ Date: _____ Time: _____.

APPENDIX D

ALCOHOL DETOXIFICATION PROTOCOL # 3

Patient Name: _____   *ID#:*_____

56. Admit to:
57. Regular Diet
58. Vital signs per policy
59. Administer 0.1 cubic centimeters intradermally to left forearm Tuberculin Purified Protein Derivative; repeat in two weeks when applicable.
60. Multivitamins one tab orally daily for length of stay
61. Thiamine 100 milligrams orally twice daily for 5 days, then
62. Thiamine 100 milligrams orally once daily thereafter for length of stay
63. Librium 75 milligrams orally as initial dose then
64. Librium 75 milligrams orally every 6 hours for 24 hours, then
65. Librium 50 milligrams orally every 6 hours for 24 hours, then
66. Librium 35 milligrams orally every 6 hours for 24 hours, then
67. Librium 25 milligrams orally every 6 hours for 24 hours, then
68. Librium 10 milligrams orally every 6 hours for 24 hours, then discontinue
69. Librium 25 milligrams orally every 4 hours as needed based on signs and symptoms of withdrawal for 5 days, then discontinue
70. Levsin 0.125 milligrams sublingually every 6 hours as needed for abdominal cramps for 5 days

71. Vistaril 50 milligrams orally every 4 hours as needed for anxiety or agitation for length of stay
72. 48 hours after discontinuation of the detoxification protocol Campral 333 milligrams, (2 tablets) will be initiated orally three times per day
73. Trazodone 50 milligrams orally at bed time as needed for insomnia for length of stay
74. May repeat Trazodone 50 milligrams orally 1 additional dose 2 hours after the first dose if the first dose is not effective as needed for insomnia for length of stay
75. Clonidine 0.2 milligrams orally now, then
76. Clonidine 0.1 milligrams orally every 6 hours for 24 hours, then
77. Clonidine 0.1 milligrams orally every 8 hours for 24 hours, then
78. Clonidine 0.1 milligrams orally every 12 hours for 24 hours, then discontinue
79. Hold Clonidine if systolic blood pressure is less than100 and/or heart rate is less than 50
80. Tegretol 200 milligrams orally twice daily for length of stay
81. Serum Tegretol Level in 5 days
82. Milk of Magnesia 30 cubic centimeters orally twice daily as needed for constipation for length of stay
83. Kaopectate 30 cubic centimeters orally twice daily as needed for diarrhea for length of stay
84. Tylenol ii tabs orally three times a day as needed for headache or temp above 101° F for length of stay
85. Motrin 600 milligrams orally every 6 hours as needed for muscle aches or pain for length of stay
86. Robitussin 10 milliliters orally every 4 hours as needed for cough for length of stay
87. Cepacol throat lozenges one orally every 4 hours as needed for sore throat for length of stay
88. Random Urine Drug Screen (as determined by nursing)
89. Complete the CIWA (for alcohol) if considering administration of PRN detox medication.

Routine Labs: ____ CBC   ____ SMAC   ____Urinalysis   ____Serum Pregnancy Test

____ Urine Pregnancy Test   ____Urine Drug Screen

Physician/APN Signature: _____ Date: _____ Time: _____

NOTE: This protocol may be adjusted at any time by the Medical Staff.

REFERENCES

1. Substance Abuse and Mental Health Services Administration (SAMHSA), Office of Applied Studies. National Household Survey on Drug Abuse: volume 1. 2001 Summary of National Findings. Rockville (MD): DHHS Publication; 2002. NHSDA Series H-17, DHHS Publication. No. SMA 02–3758.
2. Office of National Drug Control Policy. The economic costs of drug abuse in the United States, 1992-1998. Washington, DC: Executive Office of the President; 2001 (Publication No. NCJ-190636).
3. McGinnis JM, Foege WH. Actual causes of death in the United States. J Am Med Assoc 1993;270:2207–12.

4. Hupkens C, Knibbe R, Drop M. Alcohol consumption in the European community: Uniformity and diversity in drinking patterns. Addiction 1993;88:1391–404.
5. Phillips S, Haycock C, Boyle D. Development of an alcohol withdrawal for protocol: CNS collaborative exemplar. Clin Nurse Spec 2006;20(4):190–8.
6. Naegle MA, D'Avanzo CE. Addictions & substance abuse: strategies for advanced practice nursing. Upper Saddle River (NJ): Prentice Hall Health; 2001.
7. Nadelmann E. Caps across orders: the Internationalization of U.S. criminal law enforcement. University Park (PA): Pennsylvania State University Press; 1993.
8. Lejoyeux M, Solomon J, Ades J. Benzodiazepine treatment for alcohol-dependent patients. Alcohol Alcohol 1998;33(6):563–75.
9. Nimmerrichter AA, Walter H, Gutierrez-Lobos KE, et al. Double-blind controlled trial of hydroxybutyrate and clomethiazole in the treatment of alcohol withdrawal. Alcohol Alcohol 2002;37(1):67–73.
10. Streeton C, Whelan G. Naltrexone, a relapse prevention maintenance treatment of alcohol dependence: a meta-analysis of randomized control trials. Alcohol Alcohol 2001;36(6):544–52.
11. Ott PJ, Tarter RE, Ammerman RT. Sourcebook on substance abuse: etiology, epidemiology, assessment and treatment. Boston: Allyn and Bacon; 1999.
12. Brown B. Use of alcohol by addict and non-addict populations. Am J Psychol 1973;130:599–601.
13. Liebson I, Bigelow G, Flamer R. Alcoholism among methadone patients: A specific treatment method. American Journal of Psychiatry 1973;130:483–5.
14. El-Bassel N, Shilling RF, Turnbull JE, et al. Correlates of alcohol use among methadone patients. Alcohol Clin Exp Res 1993;17:681–6.
15. Caputo F, Addolorato G, Domenicali M, et al. Short-term methadone administration reduces alcohol consumption in non-alcoholic heroin addicts. Alcohol Alcohol 2002;37(2):164–8.

Underage Drinking
An Evolutionary Concept Analysis

Sandra N. Jones, DrNP, APRN, PMHCNS-BC[a],*,
Roberta L. Waite, EdD, APRN, CNS-BC[b,c]

KEYWORDS

- Underage drinking • Alcohol • Adolescents • Research • Policy • Ethics

KEY POINTS

- Underage drinking is a major cause of morbidity and mortality for American youths and young adults.
- Negative consequences of underage drinking range from academic problems to intentional and unintentional injuries, acts directed toward self or others, and death.
- Nurses, regardless of practice settings, are on the frontline of defense.
- The take-home message is to delay/deter the first drink of alcohol.

INTRODUCTION

According to the Office of the Surgeon General, the most widely abused substance by American youths is alcohol.[1] Adverse outcomes of underage drinking (alcohol consumption by those younger than 21 years) contribute to the morbidity and mortality of American youth and young adults as well as contribute to serious personal, social, and economic consequences for youths, their families, communities, and the society. The purpose of this article is threefold: (1) to present the findings of the state-of-the-art usage of the concept underage drinking that illustrate the morbidity and mortality aspects of underage drinking, (2) to present implications for nurses for how to address underage drinking across practice settings, and (3) to bring forth a message from the former Acting Surgeon General Moritsugu, which says: "A National commitment to solving the National problem of underage drinking is needed. We owe nothing less

Disclosures: None.
[a] College of Nursing and Health Professions, Drexel University, 4705 Belle Forte Road, Philadelphia, PA 19102, USA; [b] Evaluation of Community Programs, College of Nursing and Health Professions, Drexel University, Philadelphia, PA 19102, USA; [c] Interdisciplinary Research Unit, Doctoral Nursing Department, College of Nursing and Health Professions, Drexel University, Philadelphia, PA 19102, USA
* Corresponding author.
E-mail address: clinicalscholar@yahoo.com

Nurs Clin N Am 48 (2013) 401–413
http://dx.doi.org/10.1016/j.cnur.2013.05.004   nursing.theclinics.com
0029-6465/13/$ – see front matter © 2013 Elsevier Inc. All rights reserved.

to our children and our country."[1](pvii) An evolutionary concept analysis method is used to collect data, interpret the findings, and to identify areas for future research.[2] The presented evolutionary concept analysis of the concept of underage drinking serves as *a nursing response* to the Surgeon General's call to action to prevent and reduce underage drinking.

The all-encompassing nature of underage drinking and the emerging animal studies, magnetic resonance imaging (MRI), and use of positron emission tomography (PET) images have identified the impact of alcohol on the anatomic regions and functions of the developing adolescent brain. In response to these findings, *The Surgeon General's Call to Action to Prevent and Reduce Underage Drinking 2007* plan was developed.[1] The report provides a comprehensive action plan designed to foster prevention and intervention strategies for underage drinking.

RODGERS AND KNAFL'S EVOLUTIONARY CONCEPT ANALYSIS METHOD

According to Rodgers and Knafl,[2] an evolutionary concept analysis method is a systematic, inductive approach to knowledge development. Rodgers and Knafl's methodology is described in detail elsewhere.[3] The methodology involves the development of 7 primary activities, which include (1) identifying the concept of interest, (2) choosing the setting and sample, (3) collecting and managing the data, (4) analyzing the data, (5) identifying an exemplar, (6) interpreting the results, and (7) identifying the implications (4). These activities are operationalized by examining the state-of-the-art usage of the concept of underage drinking.

Activity: Identifying the Concept of Interest and Associated Expressions

Rodgers and Knafl[4] describe this activity as identifying "the concept of interest and appropriate expressions."[4](p85) The concept of underage drinking is the concept of interest for this evolutionary concept analysis. The National Minimum Drinking Age Act of 1984 set the legal minimum drinking age at 21 years.[5] Both the Centers for Disease Control and Prevention (CDC)[6] and Healthy People 2010[7] describe underage drinking as a preventable priority health-risk behavior contributing to the leading causes of morbidity and mortality among American youths and young adults.

Surrogate terms

Across the literature, the term *underage drinking* is often used interchangeably (even in the same report or article) with surrogate terms, such as *underage alcoholism*, *underage alcohol use*, *adolescent alcohol use*, *underage alcohol consumption*, *adolescent substance use*, *underage drinkers*, *adolescent risk behavior*, *drinking behavior*.

Concepts related to the concept of underage drinking

A review of the literature identified the following related concepts: alcohol overdose (AOD), driving under the influence (DUI), and riding with drinking drivers (RWDD).[8] The National Highway Traffic Safety Administration (NHTSA) views AOD as a national phenomenon, which places underage drinkers at a high risk for adverse outcomes, such as fatal alcohol-related crashes.[8]

Activity: Identifying the Appropriate Setting and Sample

Rodgers and Knafl[4] define the setting as "the time period to be examined and the disciplines or types of literature to be included."[4](pp87) Publications were selected from English-language literature that crossed the disciplines of medicine, psychology, nursing, and education. In addition, data are obtained from specialty addictions journals and the review of seminal publications and government Web sites. The population of interest is American youth from 4th to 12th grade. The time frame under examination is 2000 to 2012.

Activity: Collecting and Managing the Data

Rodgers and Knafl view this activity as "an inductive, discovery approach…focuses on the collection and analysis of raw data."[4(p90)] Searches of MEDLINE, PsycINFO, CINAH (Cumulative Index to Nursing and Allied Health), ERIC (Education Resources Information Center), and Social Work Search are conducted in accordance with Rodgers and Knafl's guidelines.[4] In each database, the keyword *underage drinking* is cross-referenced with *alcohol*, *adolescents*, *research*, *policy*, and *ethics*. In addition, seminal publications were obtained from governmental agencies, specialty groups, and nursing literature. In all, a total of 56 publications were included in the analysis to examine the current state-of-the-art usage of the concept underage drinking.

Activity: Analyzing the Data by Identifying Major Themes and Attributes

Rodgers and Knafl[4] describe this activity as the examination of the literature to identify major themes organizing and labeling the major attributes of the concept. Twelve major themes and attributes contributing to the current state-of-the-art usage of the concept underage drinking include (1) legality and ethics, (2) economics, (3) morbidity, (4) mortality, (5) alcohol consumption, (6) parental attitudes/peers, (7) age of initiation, (8) gender differences, (9) environment, (10) risk/protective factors, (11) negative consequences, and (12) alcohol/adolescent brain (**Fig. 1**). The presentation of the themes and attributes of the concept underage drinking follows.

Attribute: legality and ethics of underage drinking

Public Policy led to the development of federal laws addressing the issue of underage drinking. The National Minimum Drinking Age Act of 1984 required all states to set 21 years as the legal age for the purchase or public possession of alcoholic beverages.[5] Specified circumstances were delineated under which the public possession of alcohol beverages by underage drinkers is legally permitted, for example, established religious purposes. State level laws vary across states in terms of possession of alcohol, with whom, the type of, and whether or not the underage drinker can consume alcohol.[5] Overall, minimum age drinking laws are viewed as effective deterrents to the overall rate of underage drinking and driving.[1,5,8,9]

Since 2008, a national debate has emerged over the question of reducing the minimal legal drinking age from 21 years to 18 years.[3,9] Strong supporters of reducing the minimum legal drinking age laws to 18 years are the Amethyst Initiative and Choose Responsibility organizations. However, organizations like the NHTSA and Mothers Against Drunk Driving staunchly support keeping the minimum legal drinking age (MLDA) at 21 years.[3,9] Fell[9] provides evidence that there is an inverse relationship between MLDA laws and alcohol-related traffic crashes. When the MLDA increases to 21 years of age, the number of alcohol-related traffic crashes decrease, and alcohol-related traffic fatalities increase when MLDA laws are reduced to 18 years of age.[9] Jones and Lachman developed ethical considerations of reducing MLDA laws 18 years of age.[3] The investigators call attention to both sides of the issue and are supportive of the current MLDA of 21 years.[3] Jones and Lachman write the following:

The argument that young adults have the privilege or right to drink alcohol at age 18 may be argued from the principle of autonomy. Many argue to allow people to have control over themselves and to be able to make decisions in their lives. It is the right to self-determination. It is true that respect for autonomy is the weightiest of moral principles. However, by allowing young persons to learn how to drink alcohol in

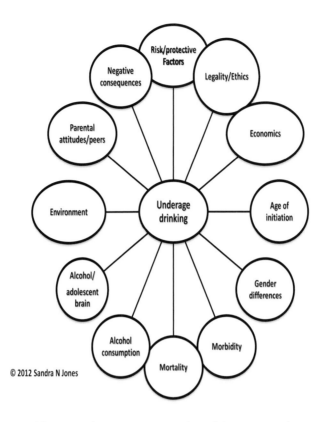

Derived from an Evolutionary Concept Analysis of the Concept Underage Drinking

Fig. 1. Major themes and attributes of underage drinking. (*Courtesy of* Sandra N. Jones, Philadelphia, PA.)

bars, which are not controlled, supervised environments, are we not putting them in harm's way? We owe them a duty of nonmaleficence, and we owe the other drivers and passengers on the road the best evidence-based decision on this issue.[3(p141)]

Attribute: economics

A study by Miller and colleagues[10] in 2005 estimated the economical costs of underage drinking as $61.9 billion. These costs included direct health care costs totaling $5.4 billion, $14.9 billion in loss work productivity, and $41.6 billion in lost quality of life.[10]

Attribute: morbidity

In this evolutionary concept analysis, the lead author describes the morbidity of underage drinking in terms of alcohol consumption, incidence and prevalence, and the short-term and long-term physical and psychological effects of alcohol. The Office of Applied Statistics defined a drink as "a can or bottle of beer, a glass of wine or a wine cooler, a shot of liquor, or a mixed drink with liquor in it"[11(p24)]; a sip or two from a drink is not viewed as alcohol consumption.[11] The National Institute on Alcohol Abuse and Alcoholism defines a standard drink: "A standard drink is any drink that contains about 14 g of pure alcohol (about 0.6 fluid ounces or 1.2 tablespoons)."[12(pp1)] Levels of alcohol consumption are described as the following: (1) current (past month) use is at least one drink in the past 30 days (includes binge and heavy use), (2) binge use is 5 or more drinks on the same occasion at least 1 day in the past 30 days, and (3) heavy use is 5 or more drinks on the same occasion on each of 5 or more days in the past 30 days.[6,11]

The Center for Substance Abuse Research reported the incidence of underage drinking as 7970 American youths, daily, (aged 12–17 years) drank alcohol for the first time.[13] Further illustrating the incidence of underage drinking is the news that 4.3 million recent alcohol initiates were younger than 21 years at the time of initiation.[13] Data describing the prevalence of alcohol use are generally presented in terms of life-time, annual, 30-day, current use, and daily prevalence.[14] Based on self-reports of 7.2 million youths aged 12 to 20 years, the 2006 National Survey on Drug Use and Health indicated prevalence rates of current alcohol use as 3.9% among persons aged 12 or 13 years, 15.6% of persons aged 14 or 15 years, 29.7% of 16 or 17 year olds, and 51.6% of those aged 18 to 20 years (**Fig. 2**).[14] However, an understudied aspect of underage drinking is alcohol use by youths aged 12 years and younger.[15,16] The PRIDE Surveys administer national surveys that measured alcohol use in elementary school-aged children (youths younger than 12 years); their findings revealed a national average of 6.9% of fourth graders, 8.6% of fifth graders, and 12.9% of sixth graders who reported alcohol use within the past year.[16]

Immediate physical effects of alcohol are dose related and to an extent related to the physical characteristics of the individual, with symptoms ranging from dizziness to loss of balance and talkativeness.[12] In low to moderate amounts of alcohol con-sumption, symptoms entail slurred speech, blurred vision, disturbed sleep, nausea and vomiting, headache, thirst, dizziness, and fatigue.[12] Short-term psychological effects of alcohol consumption may produce symptoms, such as decreased inhibi-tions, impaired memory, and impaired decision-making skills, which may lead to harmful behavior directed toward self and/or others.[12]

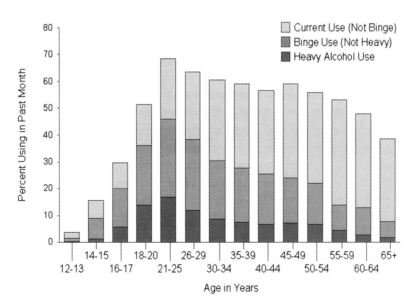

Fig. 2. Current, binge, and heavy alcohol use among persons aged 12 years or older, by age (2006). (*From* Substance Abuse and Mental Health Services Administration. (2010). Results from the 2009 National Survey on Drug Use and Health: Volume I. Summary of National Find-ings (Office of Applied Studies, NSDUH Series H-38A, HHS Publication No. SMA 10-4856 Find-ings). Rockville, MD. Available at: http://www.samhsa.gov/data/2k9/2k9Resultsweb/web/2k9results.htm. Accessed January 30, 2013.)

Long-term physical and psychological effects of alcohol consumption include medical issues, including lung and cardiovascular disease, stroke, cancer, human immunodeficiency virus/AIDS, hepatitis B and C, lung disease, alcohol abuse, alcohol dependence, and impaired brain functioning.[17]

According to the American Psychiatric Association, alcohol abuse is defined as "a maladaptive pattern of abuse use… occurring within a 12-month period"[18(p199)] that lead to malfunctioning in major role duties, alcohol use in perilous situations, legal problems that are alcohol related, and impairment of interpersonal relationships.[18] Alcoholism, also known as alcohol dependence, is defined as a debilitating disease characterized by 4 symptoms: craving, loss of control when drinking, physical dependence on alcohol, and tolerance requiring the need to drink greater amounts of alcohol despite persistent or recurrent social or interpersonal problems.[18]

Attribute: mortality

Motor vehicle crashes are the leading cause of death for underage drivers (aged 15–20 years).[5] Subsequently, much attention has been devoted to the examination of underage drinking and alcohol-related injury and fatal car crashes.[5,8,9] According to Grube and Voas,[19] DUI and RWDD can be predicted by the expectancies and normative beliefs of the adolescent. Exemplars include expectancies of physical risks resulting from DUI, the extent of disapproval by peers, and the enforcement of DUI.[19] In 2004, the NHTSA reported 3620 drivers aged 15 to 20 years were killed in fatal crashes, with an additional 303 000 injured.[8] The NHTSA reports that between 1994 and 2004, underage drivers (aged 15–20 years) accounted for 6.3% (12.4 million) of all drivers involved in fatal crashes.[8] Also, 26% of underage male drivers had been drinking at the time of a fatal crash as compared with 12% of underage female drivers involved in fatal crashes.[8] The NHTSA also reported that, in 2004, a total of 300 underage drinkers who were motorcycle operators (aged 15–20 years) were killed in fatal crashes and 8000 were injured.[8]

The Remove Intoxicated Drivers organization estimated that as many as 4000 deaths occur annually from alcohol overdosing.[20] Alcohol poisoning depresses the central nervous system. Alcohol poisoning results from an overdose of alcohol, which is dependent upon several factors such as body habitués, the amount of alcohol consumed, an individual's metabolic rate and other factors. Effects stemming from this cause breathing to stop, resulting in death or the possibility of irreversible brain damage. Signs of this dangerous condition can include mental confusion, stupor, coma or the person cannot be roused, vomiting, slow or irregular breathing, hypothermia or low body temperature, and bluish or pale skin.[21]

Attribute: negative consequences

The CDC reports that negative consequences of underage drinking include problems with academic achievement, absenteeism, lateness; participation in violent activities or the recipient of violent acts, decreased participation in age appropriate activities; and legal difficulties due to violent acts and drinking and driving.[6] Additional adversities stemming from underage drinking include physical problems (e.g. brain impairment), undesired or forced sexual intercourse and unprotected sexual activity, unplanned pregnancy, increased risk for suicide and homicide, and poly substance abuse.[6] Adding to the negative consequences of underage drinking is the development of alcohol as a gateway drug to illicit substance usage. Kandel and colleagues[22] describe the gateway process as stages of progression in drug involvement that follow a specific sequential pattern, from the use of tobacco or alcohol to the use of illicit drugs other than marijuana.[22]

Attribute: alcohol pathways for underage drinkers

Adolescence is viewed as a high-risk developmental time of vulnerability to alcohol use and its negative consequences.[1] Based on the review of the literature, the lead author identified 3 pathways for underage drinkers, not all inclusive (**Fig. 3**): (1) Pathway one is nondrinkers except for a few sips. Findings from the national *2011 Youth Risk Behavior Survey* revealed 33.3% of a representative sample of American high school students had never had a drink of alcohol other than a few sips.[23] (2) Pathway two is experimentation with alcohol. The Academy of Child and Adolescent Psychiatry states: "Experimentation with alcohol and drugs during adolescence is common…Some teens will experiment and stop, or continue to use occasionally, without significant problems."[24(p1)] (3) Pathway three is alcohol dependency. The Academy of Child and Adolescent Psychiatry states that some adolescents "will develop a dependency, moving on to more dangerous drugs and causing significant harm to themselves and possibly others… it is difficult to know which teens will experiment and stop and which will develop serious problems."[24(p1)] According to the National Institute on Drug Abuse (NIDA), no single factor determines whether a person will become addicted to alcohol/drugs.[17]

Attribute: influence of alcohol on the developing adolescent brain

Giedd's[25] studies reveal the prefrontal cortex lobes of the adolescent brain continue to develop into the 20s, thereby lengthening the period of time the brain is exposed to the harmful effects of alcohol. What are these harmful effects? First, the frontal cortex is the thinking center of the brain; it powers our ability to think, plan, solve problems, and make decisions.[17] Drug and alcohol abuse can disrupt the development of these critical functions.[17] Second, the limbic system contains the brain's reward circuit; it links together several brain structures that control and regulate an individual's ability to feel pleasure.[17] Feeling pleasure motivates us to repeat behaviors, such as eating, which are actions that are critical to our existence. The limbic system is activated when we perform these activities and when engaging in illicit drug usage.[17] Most drugs of abuse directly or indirectly target the brain's reward system by flooding the circuit with dopamine.[17] Dopamine is a neurotransmitter present in regions of the brain that regulate movement, emotion, cognition, motivation, and feelings of pleasure.[17]

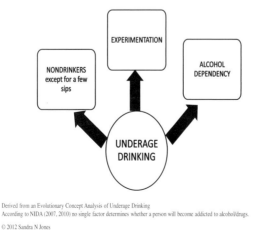

Derived from an Evolutionary Concept Analysis of Underage Drinking
According to NIDA (2007, 2010) no single factor determines whether a person will become addicted to alcohol/drugs.

© 2012 Sandra N Jones

Fig. 3. Alcohol pathways for underage drinkers. (*Courtesy of* Sandra N. Jones, Philadelphia, PA.)

The overstimulation of this system, which rewards our natural behaviors, produces the euphoric effects sought by people who abuse drugs and teaches them to repeat the behavior. It is the repeated use of alcohol and drugs that can lead to alcohol/drug dependency. According to the NIDA, no single factor determines whether a person will become addicted to alcohol/drugs.[17] The overall risk for the development of alcohol dependence is influenced by the number of risk factors (eg, biologic makeup of the individual [gender or ethnicity]; the developmental stage of the adolescent and their environment; and the number of protective factors).[17]

Attribute: risk and protective factors of underage drinking
An in-depth discussion of the risks and protective factors of underage drinking is beyond the scope of this article. However, examples of risk factors are provided: a family history of alcohol abuse, parents with antisocial behavior, parental maltreatment, neglect and poor parental supervision, risk-taking behavior, underage smoking and illicit drug use, childhood attention deficit problems, psychological and psychiatric impairment of the child or mother, parental influence, residing in the inner-city environment, and exposure to a drug-culture environment.[17,26,27] An example of the protective action of the federal government is provided. Laws exist in all 50 states against underage drinking with the minimum purchase age for alcohol set at 21 years.[5] Fell[9] reports the MLDA laws have reduced alcohol-related traffic fatalities among 18- to 20-year-old drivers by 13% and have saved an estimated 23,733 lives since 1975.[11] The NIDA identified risk and protective factors across individual, family, peer, school, and community domains.[17]

Attribute: influence of the environment
The influence of the urban school environment and of the urban neighborhood as a primary socialization experience is an understudied area in minority adolescent populations that warrants attention.[25–27] Centers and Weist[27] and Goddard[26] examined the impact of drug dealing on inner-city adolescents and called for efforts at all levels to address the phenomenon. Lambert and colleagues[28] examined the association of perceived neighborhood disorganization and subsequent substance use among African American adolescents and stressed the significance of contextual neighborhood variables in the development of substance use in this population. While examining the effects of alcohol advertising and marketing on adolescent alcohol-related beliefs, a significant negative impact on youth and adult expectations and attitudes is noted. For example, Stacy and colleagues[29] report seventh graders who viewed an increased number of television programs containing alcohol commercials were more likely in the eighth grade to drink beer, wine/liquor, or to drink 3 or more drinks on at least one occasion 30 days before the follow-up survey.[29] However, Austin and colleagues[30] state the influence of underage drinking is underestimated by traditional exposure-and-effects analyses.

Attribute: gender differences
Results from the 2006 National Survey on Drug Use and Health, based on self-reports from respondents aged 12 to 20 years, indicated gender differences exist among underage drinkers.[14] The survey revealed 29.2% of the boys as compared with 27.4% of the girls reported current alcohol use. Differences in alcohol consumption were also noted between adolescents and adults.[1] Although youths between the ages of 12 and 20 years drink less frequently than adults (6 occasions a month), they consume more alcohol. On average, they consume 5 drinks per occasion, as compared with adult men who consume 5 or more drinks per occasion and adult women who consume 4 or more drinks per occasion.[1]

Attribute: age of first use

The reported age of the first use of alcohol varied in terminology and definitions across the literature and is generally reported in age categories, such as younger than 12 years or older than 12 years. For example, the National Survey on Drug Use and Health reports the average age for the first use of alcohol among persons aged 12 to 49 years as 18.7 years.[14] The *Surgeon General Call to Action to Prevent and Reduce Underage Drinking* report identified the age of the first use of alcohol as follows: "by age 15, approximately 50% of boys and girls have had a whole drink of alcohol; by age 21, approximately 90% have done so."[1(p3)] Lastly, the CDC reported the age of the first use: "Nationwide, 25.6% of students had drunk alcohol (other than a few sips) for the first time before age 13 years."[6(p17)] Hawkins and colleagues[31] reported a strong association between ingestion of alcohol at an early age and a higher level of underage drinking reported at 17 to 18 years of age. Even so, a dearth of research is noted in the study of underage drinking for youths aged 12 years. Donovan and colleagues[15] described self-reports of early underage drinking by third and fourth graders as reliable and valid and calls for the study of variables related to underage drinking in populations aged 12 years and younger.

Attribute: parental attitude/peers

The Surgeon General points out: "adolescent alcohol use is not an acceptable rite of passage but a serious threat to adolescent development and health."[1(pvii)] Research has found that parental attitudes toward underage drinking and parental alcohol-related behavior may serve as a risk factor or as a protective factor for underage drinking.[32] Yu[32] also described parental attitudes toward alcohol as a risk factor when parental alcohol use through extensive interaction increases the risk of underage drinking; however, Yu viewed parental control of alcohol consumption in the home as a protective factor that reduces the likelihood of underage drinking.[32] The influence of the home environment is usually most important in childhood. Parents or older family members who abuse alcohol or drugs, or who engage in criminal behavior, can increase children's risks of developing their own drug problems.[17] Friends and acquaintances have the greatest influence during adolescence. Drug-abusing peers can sway even those without risk factors to try drugs for the first time.[17]

Activity: Interpreting the Results to Reflect Currant Usage of the Concept Underage Drinking

Utilization of Rodgers and Knafl's[2] evolutionary concept analysis method to determine the current state-of-art usage of the concept of underage drinking revealed a general consensus that underage drinking is a complex, multifaceted national health problem. Twelve major themes and attributes were identified in this analysis: risk/protective factors, legality/ethics, economics, age of initiation, gender differences, morbidity, mortality, alcohol consumption, environment, parental attitudes/peers, alcohol and the adolescent brain, and negative consequences of underage drinking (see **Fig. 2**). Attributes of the concept of underage drinking are biopsychosocial in nature and affect the individual, family, community, and the society. The economic costs of underage drinking, both direct and indirect, total in the billions of dollars annually. Yet, how does one ethically measure in dollars the lost of a loved one? How does one measure in dollars the quality of life for the underage drinker, the family, and the community afflicted with problem of underage drinking? The extensive negative consequences of underage drinking spanning from poor academic performance to death necessitate sophisticated primary, secondary, and tertiary interventions by members of the health care team.

Health care providers, specifically nurses, are positioned well to effectively address many of these concerns. There is an emerging trend to view underage drinking from a lifespan developmental perspective, which in turn facilitates a holistic approach to prevention and treatment strategies. Results from emerging MRI studies, alcohol-related animal studies, and PET studies have directed a focus to the developing adolescent brain and the alcohol-related damage. Nonetheless, there remains a paucity of studies that examine the phenomenon of underage drinking by youths aged 12 years and younger.

Activity: Identify Exemplar Case

According to Rodgers and Knafl,[4] the goal of this activity is to "illustrate the characteristics of the concept in relevant contexts."[4(p96)] The following case model of the concept of underage drinking is based on a real-life clinical case drawn from the lead author's clinical practice. A 12-year-old sixth-grade student (J) is exposed to his peers' alcohol consumption on a daily basis. Provided with the opportunity to consume alcohol beverages, J thinks underage drinking is acceptable behavior and a rite of passage for the American adolescent. As an added risk factor, J's mother is diagnosed with alcohol dependence. The risk factors surrounding J (opportunity, accessibility, peer pressure, and an alcohol-dependent mother) place J at a high risk to initiate the first use of alcohol. J finally drinks a 40-oz beer at 13 years of age (age of first use). He enjoyed the immediate short-term effects (the buzz) and shortly thereafter begins to consume beer in large amounts on a daily basis.

The consequences of this case are that by 15 years of age, the student experienced poor school attendance and extensive absenteeism from school (alcohol abuse). By 19 years of age, the student is diagnosed with alcohol dependency and is frequently revolving in and out of treatment centers and hospitalization for alcohol-related problems. He now requires consumption of larger amounts of alcohol to deter alcohol withdrawal and to achieve the desired effects (the buzz). By 20 years of age, the student is involved in a fatal traffic crash driving while under the influence alcohol (mortality).

Activity: Identify Hypotheses and Implications for Further Developments

Continued research is needed to study the complex variables involved in underage drinking by youths 12 years and younger in terms of developing effective prevention and intervention strategies.[1] As a clinical scientist in training, concerned about underage drinking, the lead author poses critical research questions: What are the antecedents of underage drinking by youths aged 12 years and younger living in an urban neighborhood? Is there a difference in school violence behaviors among students reporting their first drink of alcohol at 12 years of age and younger and students reporting the age of their first drink of alcohol at 13 years and older? What role does spirituality play on underage drinking?

IMPLICATIONS FOR NURSES ACROSS PRACTICE SETTINGS

The American Nurses Association's Code of Ethics, Provision 8.2 states that nurses have a responsibility to become knowledgeable about issues influencing the health of their populations.[33] At the very least, the nurse can become informed about the problem of underage drinking and assess how it affects the population for which they provide care. At the very least, regardless of practice settings, nurses can begin to dialogue with other nurses and team members about the problem of underage drinking. Nurses can play an important role in educating youth, families, and other concerned individuals about the risk/protective factors and negative consequences of underage drinking. Nurses can become active advocates in the community by supporting the MLDA laws at 21 years of age. We can join our local school boards to educate and develop school policies. Foremost, nurses have the skills to conduct primary, secondary, and tertiary interventions, such as screening, assessment, treatment, referral, development of health policies, and conducting research.

Reading relevant peer-reviewed articles and/or books by expert addictions nurses for nurses, such as *Nursing Care of the Addicted Client* by Allen, is advised.[34] Although this book is dated, the basic content remains largely relevant addressing the following: theoretical perspectives of addictions nursing practice, maternal-child nursing, prevention, screening and detection, assessment and diagnosis, interventions and treatment, and addictions nursing research. Numerous tools are available for the screening and assessment of drugs and alcohol use, such as Cage and Cage-Aid, T-Ace Questions, and the TWEAK TEST.[34] The Screening, Brief Intervention, and Referral to Treatment (SBIRT) program is a comprehensive approach to early intervention and treatment of alcohol and other drug-use problems.[35] SBIRT training addresses the early identification and referral of at-risk alcohol and drug users. Nurse administrators and nurse educators can institute and promote the SBIRT training for nurses across practice settings. Yet another tool of practical use is the CRAFTT tool, which is developed to screen adolescents for alcohol and other drug-use problems.[36]

SUMMARY

Rodger and Knafl's[2] evolutionary concept analysis method proved to be an effective contemporary approach in the development of the current state-of-the-art usage of the concept of underage drinking. Twelve themes and attributes were identified: (1) legality and ethics, (2) economics, (3) morbidity, (4) mortality, (5) alcohol consumption, (6) parental attitudes/peers, (7) age of initiation, (8) gender differences, (9) environment, (10) risk/protective factors, (11) negative consequences, and (12) alcohol and the adolescent (see **Fig. 1**). Evidence from the evolutionary concept analysis of underage drinking revealed the enormous scope of the concept of underage drinking whose characteristics are human-bound, dynamic in nature, contextually dependent, and contain practical utility.[2] Underage drinking is viewed as a major cause of morbidity and mortality of the nations' youth and a destroyer of quality of life for many. The negative consequences of underage drinking range from academic problems to intentional and unintentional injuries, acts directed toward self or others, alcohol dependency/alcoholism as early as 18 years of age, and death. Nurses on the frontline of health care are aptly positioned to provide the needed interventions. This evolutionary concept analysis of the current state-of-the-art usage of the concept of underage drinking is offered *as a nursing response* to the Surgeon General's call to action to reduce and prevent underage drinking. The take-home message is this: delay/deter the first drink of alcohol.

REFERENCES

1. Department of Health and Human Services (DHHS). The Surgeon General's call to action to prevent and reduce underage drinking. U.S. Department of Health and Human Services, Office of the Surgeon General; 2007. p. vii. Available at: http://www.surgeongeneral.gov. Accessed September 10, 2008.
2. Rodgers B, Knafl K. Concept development in nursing: foundations, techniques and applications. Philadelphia: WB Saunders Company; 1993, 2003.
3. Jones SN, Lachman VD. Continuing the dialogue: reducing the minimum legal drinking age law from age 21 to 18. J Addict Nurs 2011;22:138–43. http://dx.doi.org/10.3109/10884602.2011.585724.

4. Rodgers B. Concept analysis: an evolutionary view. In: Rodgers B, Knafl K, editors. Concept development in nursing: foundations, techniques and applications. 1st edition. Philadelphia: WB Saunders Company; 1993. p. 7–92.

5. The 1984 National Minimum Drinking Age Act, [23 U.S.C. § 158] 1984. Available at: http://www.alcoholpolicy.niaaa.nih.gov/index.asp?SEC=%7B9937ACFC-DB3A-4159-B068-A302CEEE0EDF%7D&Type=B_BASIC. Accessed April 23, 2008.

6. Centers for Disease Control and Prevention (CDC). Data & statistics: YRBSS youth risk behavior surveillance system. Centers for Disease Control and Prevention; 2007. Available at: http://www.cdc.gov/HealthyYouth/yrbs/index.htm. Accessed May 1, 2008.

7. Department Health and Human Services (DHHS). Healthy people 2010 midcourse review. Department Health and Human Services; 2006. Available at: http://www.healthypeople.gov/data/midcourse/html/focusareas/FA26Introduction.htm. Accessed September 9, 2007.

8. National Highway Traffic Safety Administration. Young drivers: traffic safety facts, 2004 data. National Highway Traffic Safety Administration n.d. Available at: http://wwwnrd.nhtsa.dot.gov/pdf/nrd-30/NCSA/TSF2004/809918.pdf. Accessed April 23, 2008.

9. Fell J. An examination of the criticisms of the minimum legal drinking age 21 laws in the United States from a traffic safety perspective. Pacific Institute for Research and Evaluation, National Highway Traffic Safety Administration; 2008. Available at: http://www.nhtsa.gov/staticfiles/DOT/NHTSA/Traffic%20Injury%20Control. Accessed January 30, 2009.

10. Miller T, Levy D, Spicer R, et al. Societal costs of underage drinking. J Stud Alcohol 2006;67:519–28.

11. Office of Applied Studies (OAS). The NSDUH report: alcohol dependence or abuse and age at first use. Office of Applied Studies; 2003. Available at: http://www.oas.samhsa.gov/2k4/ageDependence/ageDependence.htm. Accessed January 4, 2008.

12. National Institute on Alcohol Abuse and Alcoholism. Understanding the impact of alcohol on human health and well-being. National Institute of Health n.d. Available at: http://pubs.niaaa.nih.gov/publications/Practitioner/PocketGuide/pocket_guide2.htm#top. Accessed November 7, 2012.

13. Center for Substance Abuse Research (Cesar Fax). Nearly 8,000 youths drink alcohol for the first time on an average day; more than 4,000 use illicit drugs for the first time, vol. 16. Baltimore (MD): Center for Substance Abuse Research; 2007. p. 43.

14. Office of Applied Studies (OAS). Results from the 2005 national survey on drug use and health: national findings. Office of Applied Studies; 2006. Available at: http://oas.samhsa.gov/nsduh/2k5nsduh/2k5results.htm#High. Accessed February 2, 2008.

15. Donovan J, Leach S, Zucker R, et al. Really underage drinkers: alcohol use among elementary students. Alcohol Clin Exp Res 2004;28:341–9.

16. Pride Surveys. Pride questionnaire report for grades 4 thru 6: 2005–06 national summaries for grade 4-6. Pride Surveys 2008. Available at: http://www.pridesurveys.com/customercenter/ue05ns.pdf. Accessed May 1, 2008.

17. National Institute on Drug Abuse [NIDA]. Drugs, brains, and behavior: the science of addiction National Institutes of Health, U.S. Department of Health and Human Services; 2010. NIH Pub Number: 10-5605.

18. American Psychiatric Association. Diagnostic and statistical manual of mental disorders: test revision. 4th edition. Arlington (VA): American Psychiatric Association; 2006.

19. Grube J, Voass R. Predicting underage drinking and driving behaviors. Addiction 1996;91:1843–57.
20. RID, USA, Inc. (n. d.) Remove intoxicated drivers. Available at: http://rid-usa.org/video.htm. Accessed May 10, 2010.
21. National Institute on Alcohol Abuse and Alcoholism. Parents: help your teens party right at graduation. National Institute on Alcohol Abuse and Alcoholism; 2012. Available at: http://pubs.niaaa.nih.gov/publications/GraduationFacts/NIAAA_graduation_flyer.pdf. Accessed February 3, 2012.
22. Kandel D, Yamaguchi K, Chen K. Stages of progression in drug involvement from adolescence to adulthood: further evidence for the gateway theory. J Stud Alcohol 1992;53:447–57.
23. Centers for Disease Control and Prevention (CDC). 2011 YRBS data user's guide. Youth Risk Behavior Surveillance System (YRBSS). Centers for Disease Control and Prevention; 2011. Available at: ftp://ftp.cdc.gov/pub/data/yrbs/2011/YRBS_2011_National_User_Guide.pdf. Accessed November 3, 2012.
24. American Academy of Child & Adolescent Psychiatry. Facts for families: teens alcohol and other drugs. American Academy of Child & Adolescent Psychiatry; 2011. Available at: http://www.aacap.org/galleries/FactsForFamilies/03_teens_alcohol_and_other_drugs.pdf. Accessed November 1, 2012.
25. Giedd J. Structural magnetic resonance imaging of the adolescent brain. Ann N Y Acad Sci 2004;1021:77–85.
26. Goddard L. Background and scope of the alcohol and other drug problem. In: Goddard LL, editor. An African-centered model of prevention for American youth at high risk. Rockville (MD): US Department of Health and Human Services; 1993. p. 1–145.
27. Centers N, Weist M. Inner city youth and drug dealing: a review of the problem. J Youth Adolesc 1998;27:395–411.
28. Lambert S, Brown T, Phillips C, et al. The relationship between perceptions and neighborhood characteristics and substance use among urban African American adolescents. Am J Community Psychol 1997;34:205–18.
29. Stacy A, Zogg J, Unger J, et al. Exposure to televised alcohol ads and subsequent adolescent alcohol use. Am J Health Behav 2006;28:498–509.
30. Austin E, Chen M, Grube J. How does alcohol advertising influence underage drinking? The role of desirability, identification, and skepticism. J Adolesc Health 2006;38:376–84.
31. Hawkins J, Graham J, Maguin E, et al. Exploring the effects of age of alcohol use initiation and psychosocial risk factors on subsequent alcohol misuse. J Stud Alcohol 1997;58:280–90.
32. Yu J. The association between parental alcohol-related behaviors and children drinking. Drug Alcohol Depend 2003;69:253–62.
33. American Nurses Association. Code of ethics for nurses with interpretative statements- provision 8.2. American Nurses Association Silver; 2001. Available at: http://nursingworld.org/ethics/code/protectednwcoe813.htm#1.3. Accessed January 20, 2009.
34. Allen K. Nursing care of the addicted client. Philadelphia: Lippincott; 1996.
35. Substance Abuse and Mental Health Services Administration. Screening, brief intervention, and referral to treatment (SBIRT). Available at: http://www.samhsa.gov/prevention/sbirt/. Accessed April 10, 2012.
36. The Center for Adolescent Substance Abuse Research (CEASAR). The CRAFFT screening tool. Available at: http://www.ceasar-boston.org/CRAFFT/index.php. Accessed May 30, 2011.

Substance Use Disorders and Evidence-Based Detoxification Protocols

Albert Rundio Jr, PhD, DNP, RN, APRN, CARN-AP, NEA-BC[a,b,c,*]

KEYWORDS

- Substance use disorders • Evidence-based detoxification protocols
- Pharmacologic agents

KEY POINTS

- The role of advanced practice nursing in addictions is inclusive of the medical detoxification of patients.
- Addiction fits a biopsychosocial/spiritual disease model.
- One of the primary goals of treatment is to address the components of this model.
- Various pharmacologic agents have been used for the management of withdrawal.

INTRODUCTION/BACKGROUND INFORMATION

The impetus for this project resulted from several factors affecting advanced nursing practice in addictions. As an advanced practice nurse certified by the American Nurses Credentialing Center as an Acute Care Nurse Practitioner and an Adult Health Primary Care Nurse Practitioner as well as certified by the International Nurses Society of Addictions as a Certified Addictions Registered Nurse – Advanced Practice and licensed as a Licensed Clinical Alcohol and Drug Counselor by the Board of Marriage and Family Therapy in New Jersey, my primary area of practice for the past 11 years has been addictions.

The role of the advanced practice nurse in the facility that I practice at was conceptualized by myself and happened by circumstance rather than a well-defined plan. The Medical Director of the facility was involved in a serious car accident in 1997 and I received a telephone call both from him and the Director of Nursing requesting that I cover for him for a few days. Medical rounds had not been made for several days, and several patients needed the required history and physical examination performed as well as all other routine medical orders. I accepted the offer to be of assistance and

---

[a] College of Nursing & Health Professions, Drexel University, 1505 Race Street, Room #429, Philadelphia, PA 19102, USA; [b] International Nurses Society on Addictions, PO Box 14846, Lenexa, KS 66285-4846, USA; [c] Lighthouse at Mays Landing, 5034 Atlantic Avenue, Mays Landing, NJ 08330, USA
* College of Nursing & Health Professions, Drexel University, 1505 Race Street, Room #429, Philadelphia, PA 19102.
E-mail address: aar27@drexel.edu

Nurs Clin N Am 48 (2013) 415–436
http://dx.doi.org/10.1016/j.cnur.2013.04.002
0029-6465/13/$ – see front matter © 2013 Elsevier Inc. All rights reserved.

what evolved was full implementation of an advanced practice nursing role, thus shifting the facility from a pure medical model of care delivery to that of an advanced practice nursing model with medical oversight. The current Medical Director is supportive of the advanced practice nursing model. Our collaborative role has been to continually improve the facility and the care rendered to our patients with good quality medical and nursing care.

PATIENT POPULATION

The patient population consists of adult patients from the age of 18 years to elderly patients, although most of our patients are young adults. These patients are chemically addicted to various substances and are admitted to a residential inpatient treatment facility for detoxification from such substances. A small percentage of the patients are admitted for rehabilitation only because they have already been detoxified from substances. In this latter group, the patients self-detoxify or are detoxified at another facility before completing a residential rehabilitation program.

The treatment facility is a for-profit, private residential treatment facility located in southern New Jersey. This treatment facility is licensed by the New Jersey State Department of Health to provide acute medical detoxification of patients as well as rehabilitation services. The facility is licensed for 62 inpatient beds. There are 2 primary treatment units at this facility. The adolescent unit is licensed for 42 inpatient beds. Patients admitted to the adolescent unit are between the ages of 13 and 18 years. The adult unit is licensed for 20 inpatient beds. Fifteen of the 20 licensed adult beds are for acute medical detoxification. Five of the 20 licensed beds are for rehabilitation purposes. This treatment facility is accredited by the Joint Commission on Accreditation of Health Care Organizations. This treatment facility also has 3 intensive outpatient treatment programs. One program is housed at the treatment facility. The other 2 treatment programs are housed off site. One program is located in Ventnor, New Jersey, a border community to Atlantic City. The other outpatient program is located in Manahawkin, New Jersey, another Jersey Shore community in Ocean County, New Jersey. This project focuses only on the adult inpatient population.

INTERVENTION

The role of advanced practice nursing in addictions is inclusive of the medical detoxification of patients. Patients, when detoxified from substances, are gradually weaned down on the medication used for acute detoxification. Abrupt withdrawal of a medication could trigger acute withdrawal symptoms in patients, which could be life threatening in some circumstances.

The advanced practice role is inclusive of making daily medical and nursing rounds. Each day either the Medical Director or the advanced practice nurse had to write new orders for detoxification to wean the patient down. For example, if an alcoholic patient was on chlordiazepoxide (Librium) 50 mg every 6 hours for 24 hours, the next day, a new order had to be written that lowered the Librium dose, for example, Librium 35 mg every 6 hours for 24 hours. The advanced practice nurse questioned if there was a more efficient manner in which to detoxify patients. The suggestion was to develop medical and nursing protocols for detoxification that would be a standard order set for patients. This suggestion was supported by the Director of Nursing at the facility, because she had just had a consultant review the facility for efficiency. His recommendation was also to develop treatment protocols. With the movement toward evidence-based practice, the Medical Director fully supported this concept and charged the advanced practice nurse with the development of such protocols. A meeting was conducted with the Medical Director, the Director of Nursing, and the advanced practice nurse. It was decided that the treatment protocols should be evidence based and should incorporate current relapse prevention medications as well as the routine detoxification medications. Ten treatment protocols have been developed and implemented based on the common substances abused by patients who are admitted to this particular treatment facility. Certain abused substances, such as alcohol and opioids, have a few treatment protocols so that correct dosing of detoxification medication can be tailored to patient use and abuse patterns.

The common substances abused by the patients include the following:

- Alcohol
- Anabolic steroids
- Anxiolytics (benzodiazepines [BZDs], barbiturates)
- Amphetamines
- Club drugs (ecstasy, γ-hydroxybutyric acid [GHB], rohypnol)
- Cocaine
- Marijuana (tetrahydrocannabinol [THC])
- Nicotine
- Psychedelics/hallucinogens

Exclusion Criteria:

- Pregnant patients
- Patient with gambling addictions
- Patient with sexual addictions
- Adolescent patients (13–17 years of age)

Treatment protocols have been developed for alcohol, BZDs, and opioids. The benefits to the development of such protocols include the following:

1. Standardized written order form, which was computer generated
2. Standardized patient care protocol
3. Pharmacologic and other interventions based on current evidence in the field
4. Decrease in variation of both written orders and patient care
5. Measurement and evaluation of treatment interventions
6. Decrease in the time needed to write daily orders
7. Flexibility for change as new evidence is discovered

COMPARISON INTERVENTION/STATUS

Rather than use a comparative group with a different intervention, it was decided to implement all of the protocols at the same time, with concurrent evaluation. It was believed that the medical and nursing practitioners would be able to assess if the treatment protocols were more effective than daily handwritten orders. This theory would be assessed primarily through patient response, nursing input and feedback, and formal evaluation.

OUTCOME

Outcome evaluation consists of direct observation and qualitative evaluation, with use of a focus group of nurses.

I. Outcome evaluation
  Quantitative and qualitative evaluation with defined indicators 3 months after implementation of project

1. Direct observation of patients by nursing and medical staffs
2. Concurrent chart audit with defined indicators
   a. Number of seizures
   b. Vital signs
   c. Number of times as-needed medications are used (based on the Clinical Institute Withdrawal Assessment [CIWA] [alcohol] assessment scale)
   d. Pain Assessment Scale
   e. Number of times detoxification protocols have to be readjusted
3. Qualitative focus group of nursing staff with open-ended interview questions

CONCEPTUAL FRAMEWORK

Addiction fits a biopsychosocial/spiritual disease model. According to Ott and colleagues,[1(p175)] "it is difficult to search for single determining factors in a complex world where the individual human being is 1 biopsychosocial system." Current research in the field has reinforced the biological components of this disease process. For several years now, health practitioners have been aware that addiction is a real disease. Addicts do not elect to become addicted. With the advent of positive emission tomography (PET) scanning, brain chemistry and neurochemical transmitter release has been studied. Many receptor sites in the primitive brain area called the ventral trigeminal area have been identified, for example, opium receptors, cocaine receptors, and alcohol receptors. Some theories on addiction are that addicts may have damaged receptor sites or genetic mutations, which affect neurochemical release and saturation of receptor sites. The psychology of the individual as well as the sociologic manifestations also contribute to addiction. Spirituality has brought many individuals to recovery. It is one of the founding philosophies of 12-step programs. From my experience from performing several history and physical examinations over the years, I have observed many clients who do not relate to any spiritual entity when they are addicted.

The best way to view addiction is as a chronic disease process. This model fits addictions. Just as a diabetic may have a high blood sugar level after ingesting a large piece of cake, addicts also can relapse and turn back to substance use and abuse. Providers need to be understanding of patients who relapse, because any chronic disorder can have reoccurrences. Clinicians should not judge individuals who relapse, but rather support their recovery until it is permanent.

One of the primary goals of treatment is to address the components of this model. The biological aspect of addictions is accomplished through pharmacology both for detoxification and relapse prevention. The psychological component is addressed through psychiatric evaluation of the client, because many clients have an underlying psychiatric disorder. The social component is addressed by including the family and significant others (SOs) in the treatment process. The goal of treatment is for clients to lead an effective life, which includes returning to work or finding employment. As with any disease process, family inclusiveness is necessary, because family members can be enablers, which is contradictory to the philosophy of treatment. The spiritual component is addressed through 12-step meetings such as Alcoholics Anonymous, in which an individual's belief in a higher power is one of the founding steps in this process.

This project focused primarily on the biological aspect of this conceptual model. Ten treatment protocols were developed, implemented, and evaluated, which incorporated current evidence on pharmacologic interventions for detoxification of addicts as well as pharmacology focused on relapse prevention.

REVIEW OF THE LITERATURE
Alcohol

According to Lejoyeux and colleagues[2] and Ott and colleagues,[1] BZDs are the preferred pharmacologic agents for the treatment of acute alcohol withdrawal states. These investigators further state that mild to moderate withdrawal symptoms can be treated with BZDs on an outpatient basis, whereas severe withdrawal states require inpatient admission. Lejoyeux and colleagues[2] state that BZDs do not improve abstinence rates and in most circumstances are not indicated for long-term use. A variety of BZDs can be used for successful detoxification. Librium is the gold standard for treatment of alcohol withdrawal states. Lorazepam (Ativan) has also been used with success and is often the preferred treatment in the acute care hospital setting, because Ativan can be administered intravenously as well as orally. One of the problems with use of the BZDs is their long half-life. In some patients with liver failure secondary to cirrhosis and alcoholism, BZDs given orally are not processed quickly enough by the failing liver. Serax as an alternative BZD has been found to be more effective in these cases.

Phillips and colleagues[3] designed a process improvement project that developed an alcohol withdrawal syndrome (AWS) management protocol for the acute care hospital setting. The design of this project included a work team, which comprised physicians, pharmacists, and nurses, led by a behavioral health clinical nurse specialist. The outcome of this project was the development and integration of a safe and effective treatment protocol that effectively managed AWS. This project was facilitated by collaborative, evidence-based decision making. The investigators addressed 3 key components of care: (1) the identification of high-risk patients; (2) the initiation of prophylactic treatment; and (3) the initiation of effective and timely pharmacologic interventions in an effort to prevent medical complications in AWS, which could lead to death. The investigators also concluded from their review that BZDs are the mainstay of primary pharmacologic therapy in patients with AWS. Their preferred medication in the acute care setting was Valium (diazepam).

Nemmerrichter and colleagues[4] conducted a double-blind controlled trail of GHB and clomethiazole in the treatment of alcohol withdrawal symptoms. The purpose of the study was to assess the efficacy and safety of GHB in ameliorating symptoms of alcohol withdrawal. Patients were randomized to received either clomethiazole or GHB. One clomethiazole group was established. Two GHB groups were established, in which the dosage of GHB varied by group. The investigators concluded that there was no difference among the 3 treatment groups in the rating of alcohol withdrawal symptoms. There were also no requests for additional medication. After tapering of medication, there was no increase in withdrawal symptoms or requests for medication. This finding indicated that physical tolerance did not develop in any of the groups. The most frequently reported side effect was in the GHB group, who reported transient vertigo after the evening double dosage of medication. GHB used to be sold as a health tonic in health food stores until the potential for abuse was discovered. GHB overdose can cause a cessation of respiration, coma, and death. GHB was withdrawn from the market a few years ago. As a result of this withdrawal, GHB is usually not found in treatment protocols for alcohol dependency.

Relapse Prevention

According to Ott and colleagues,[1(p303)] "although the substitution of an abused drug with a safer controlled medication, such as methadone, for the treatment of opioid dependence has been shown to be effective, recent pharmacotherapy developments in alcohol and cocaine dependence focus more on nonsubstitution treatment (e.g. relapse prevention, reduction of craving) with medications that are not themselves habit forming."

Relapse prevention incorporates the use of other types of pharmacologic agents. Antabuse (disulfiram) has been on the market for several years now. Many clinicians have stopped prescribing Antabuse secondary to life-threatening reactions, including of death, in patients who drink alcohol when taking this medication. According to Ott and colleagues,[1] it may be an effective treatment of cocaine dependency; however, the investigators caution that further research is warranted first.

Streeton and Whelan[5] conducted a meta-analysis of naltrexone use as a relapse prevention medication for alcoholism. These investigators searched MEDLINE, EMBASE, PsychLIT, and Cochrane Controlled Trials Registry for articles published from 1976 to 2001. Their meta-analysis showed that naltrexone was superior to placebo. Patients in the naltrexone treatment groups maintained abstinence longer and had fewer episodes of relapse compared with those patients in the control groups.[5] In 2006, a pharmaceutical firm developed Vivitrol, an injectable form of naltrexone. Vivitrol is administered on a once-monthly basis and is ideal for patients who have increased liver enzymes levels, because oral naltrexone is contraindicated in such patients. Vivitrol must be ordered through the pharmaceutical firm that developed the medication and not at a standard retail pharmacy. It is important for clinicians to recognize that pharmacotherapy cannot reverse personal and social disruptions that are experienced by substance abusers, thus the need for psychosocial approaches conjointly with pharmacotherapy.

Campral (acamprosate) has also been shown to be an effective relapse prevention medication for alcoholism. Although the mechanism of action is not understood, according to Ott and colleagues,[1] the available evidence suggests that it enhances the function of N-methyl-D-aspartate, an amino acid receptor. This medication is used in treatment as a relapse prevention medication, because it improves abstinence outcome and diminishes cravings for alcohol. The standard dose of Campral is 666 mg 3 times daily administered orally.

Brown,[6] Liebson and colleagues,[7] and El-Bassel and colleagues[8] estimate that alcohol dependency rates vary from 5% to 49% among participants in methadone maintenance programs. Caputo and colleagues[9] evaluated alcohol use in nonalcoholic heroin addicts during the first 4 weeks of a treatment program. The treatment program consisted of either a methadone maintenance program or a nonmethadone maintenance program. The investigators noted that many heroin-dependent patients begin to abuse alcohol when in treatment. A total of 359 heroin-addicted patients were enrolled on an outpatient basis. All patients met the *Diagnostic and Statistical Manual of Mental Disorders, Fourth Edition* criteria. Thirty-two patients dropped out of the study. The investigators noted a significant decrease in daily alcohol intake in the methadone maintenance program compared with the nonmethadone maintenance program. The investigators concluded that the results of the study suggested a possible effect in reducing alcohol consumption by administering methadone on a short-term basis to nonalcoholic heroin-addicted patients.

Opioids

Various pharmacologic agents have been used for the management of withdrawal symptoms secondary to opioid dependency. Because opioid withdrawal consists of a constellation of flulike symptoms, including muscle aches and pains, some pharmacologic measures have included the following: muscle relaxants, methadone, L-α-acetylmethadol or levomethadyl acetate (LAAM), clonidine, phenobarbital, Symmetrel (amantadine), Librium, nonsteroidal antiinflammatory drugs, and Darvon (propoxyphene). According to Ott and colleagues,[1] LAAM is a longer-acting opioid agonist compared with methadone. The half-life of LAAM is estimated to be greater than 100 hours. After 11 years of experience in addictions nursing, I have never seen LAAM used in practice.

Withdrawal symptoms from opioids are generally not life threatening. Newer agents on the market have been used that contribute to office-based treatment of opioid dependency. According to Fiellin and colleagues,[10] the Drug Addiction Treatment Act of 2000 allowed qualifying physicians to prescribe schedule III, IV, and V narcotic medications or combinations of such medications for treating opioid-dependent patients. Buprenorphine (marketed as Subutex and Suboxone) came on the market for such office-based practice. According to Fiellin and colleagues, buprenorphine has 3 major advantages over other available alternative pharmacologic agents: (1) the medication is a partial opioid agonist, and thus, the associate withdrawal syndrome is milder; (2) the effect of this pharmacologic agent is long lasting, and thus, dosing can be limited to 2-day to 3-day intervals, reducing associate clinic visits; and (3) buprenorphine can be combined with naloxone, an opioid antagonist that blocks the effect of abuse with another opioid and also allows the medication to be administered sublingually. Ott and colleagues[1] state that naloxone does not precipitate withdrawal symptoms in those patients who have been pretreated with buprenorphine. These investigators further state that withdrawal from an 8-mg dose of buprenorphine has milder withdrawal symptoms compared with other agents and also buprenorphine creates less dependence than other medications, such as methadone.[1] Only physicians are approved to administer this medication. According to the US Food and Drug Administration (FDA), advanced practice nurses may not prescribe this medication. Some physicians have petitioned the FDA to allow prescribing of this medication by advanced practice nurses. This is an advanced practice issue confronting advanced practice nurses in addictions. Physicians who prescribe this medication must attend an 8-hour course on this pharmacologic agent. Initially, the law permitted a physician to have only 30 patients at a time in their practice. If the practice had more than 1 physician, then each physician could have 30 patients in the practice, provided that the physicians attended the 8-hour program. The law was revised, and physicians are now permitted to have up to 100 patients in their practice who are being prescribed buprenorphine.

This medication is highly regulated and physician offices are subject to surprise inspections by the Drug Enforcement Agency. Fiellin and colleagues[10] state that new patient populations have been reached with the advent of buprenorphine. The primary pharmacologic agent for relapse prevention in opioid-dependent addicts is naltrexone. Research has shown that the pharmacologic agent by itself does not contribute to long-term sobriety. Combination therapy with other modalities such as cognitive behavioral therapy and 12-step meetings contribute to longer-term sobriety. Carroll and colleagues[11] conducted a study in which contingency management (CM) (a behavioral therapy intervention) and SO involvement were evaluated as strategies to enhance treatment retention and medication compliance with naltrexone, thus contributing to longer-term sobriety. A total of 127 recently detoxified opioid-dependent patients were randomized to 1 of 3 treatment groups for a 12-week period. The groups included the following: (1) standard naltrexone treatment; (2) naltrexone treatment and CM; and (3) naltrexone treatment, CM, and SO involvement. SO involvement was described as a family member who was invited to participate in up to 6 family counseling sessions. Outcomes focused on retention in treatment, compliance with naltrexone therapy, and the number of urine specimens that were drug free. The group that had the most significant improvement outcomes was the CM group.

This group showed treatment retention and a reduction in opioid use. SO involvement did not significantly improve retention, compliance, or outcomes compared with the CM group. SO involvement was associated with improved family functioning. The investigators concluded that behavioral therapies, such as CM, are important to improve compliance with pharmacologic interventions. This study supports the notion that pharmacology alone is not sufficient, and because substance abuse is a chronic disease process, various targeted therapies must be used to adequately treat the patient.

Other Abused Substances

The literature is replete with information about other abused substances. For example, there is no relapse prevention medication for cocaine dependency, although clinical trials have investigated baclofen use in this population. Most substances are treated pharmacologically, because the patient presents with various symptoms. Most of these substances, for example, cocaine, amphetamines, club drugs, marijuana (THC), and anabolic steroids, are treated based on patients' presenting symptoms. Routine treatment protocols are generally not used in these patient populations.

Summary

PET scanning is leading the way for the clinical trials of many newer and older medications for treatment as well as relapse prevention in addicted patients. The 2 substances that the literature discusses most frequently are alcoholism and opioid dependency. Relapse pharmacologic agents are now recommended for these 2 substances when they are abused.

PROJECT DESCRIPTION

Ten detoxification treatment protocols were developed based on current evidence in the field. Three alcohol detoxification treatment protocols were developed. One BZD detoxification treatment protocol was developed. Six opioid detoxification treatment protocols were developed. Different detoxification treatment protocols for alcohol and opioid dependency were developed to curtail pharmacologic dosing with patient use and withdrawal symptom patterns. Detoxification treatment protocols included relapse prevention pharmacology, where applicable. All detoxification treatment protocols were developed by an advanced practice nurse at the treatment facility who is currently certified as a Certified Registered Nurse in Addictions Advanced Practice by the International Nurses Society on Addictions. All detoxification treatment protocols were reviewed and approved by the Medical Director at the treatment facility, who is currently board certified in addictions medicine by the American Society of Addictions Medicine and the Executive Committee at the treatment facility (equivalent to Institutional Review Board approval in other settings; see Appendix A).

After development of the detoxification treatment protocols, implementation was accomplished in the second quarter of 2008. Quantitative and qualitative evaluation with defined indicators was conducted for 3 months after implementation of project. The following indicators were monitored:

1. Direct observation of patients by nursing and medical staffs
2. Concurrent chart audit with defined indicators
   a. Number of seizures
   b. Vital signs
   c. Number of times as-needed medications are used (based on the CIWA [alcohol] assessment scale)

d. Pain Assessment Scale
e. Number of times detoxification protocols have to be readjusted
3. Qualitative focus group of nursing staff with open-ended interview questions

Outcome evaluation began with implementation of the treatment protocols for a 3-month period. Qualitative outcome research in the form of a focus group of nurses was conducted in June, 2008. All participants signed informed consent to be interviewed. Open-ended interview questions were posed. Responses were audiotaped and transcribed verbatim. Audiotapes were destroyed after transcription. A thematic analysis of the data was conducted. This study was completed in 2008. Based on this study, the detoxification protocols are reviewed, revised and updated on an annual basis.

APPENDIX A

ADULT ALCOHOL DETOXIFICATION PROTOCOL # 1
STANDING ORDERS

Patient Name: _____   **ID#:** _____

1. Admit to:
2. Regular Diet
3. Vital signs per policy
4. Administer 0.1cubic centimeters intradermally to left forearm Tuberculin Purified Protein Derivative; repeat in two weeks when applicable.
5. Multivitamins one tab orally daily for length of stay
6. Thiamine 100 milligrams orally twice daily for 5 Days, then
7. Thiamine 100 milligrams orally once daily thereafter for length of stay
8. Librium 75 milligrams orally as initial dose then
9. Librium 50 milligrams orally every 6 hours for 24 hours, then
10. Librium 35 milligrams orally every 6 hours for 24 hours, then
11. Librium 25 milligrams orally every 6 hours for 24 hours, then
12. Librium 10 milligrams orally every 6 hours for 24 hours, then discontinue
13. Librium 25 milligrams orally every 4 hours as needed based on signs and symptoms of withdrawal for 5 days
14. Levsin 0.125 milligrams sublingually every 6 hours as needed for abdominal cramps for 5 days
15. Vistaril 50 milligrams orally every 4 hours as needed for anxiety or agitation for length of stay
16. 48 hours after discontinuation of the detoxification protocol Campral 333 milligrams, (2 tablets) will be initiated orally three times per day
17. Trazadone 50 milligrams orally at bed time as needed for insomnia for length of stay
18. May repeat Trazadone 50 milligrams orally 1 additional dose 2 hours after the first dose if the first dose is not effective as needed for insomnia for length of stay
19. 48 hours after discontinuation of the detoxification protocol give Naltrexone 25 milligrams orally at bed time x 3 days then increase Naltrexone to 50 milligram once orally at bed time thereafter
20. Vivitrol 380 milligrams intramuscular to the gluteal region once monthly if patient fails Naltrexone oral challenge or if patient's liver enzymes are elevated. Notify medical staff to discuss Vivitrol therapy with the patient prior to initiation and also for written prescription.

21. Milk of Magnesia 30 cubic centimeters orally twice daily as needed for constipation for length of stay
22. Maalox 30 cubic centimeters orally twice daily as needed for indigestion for length of stay
23. Kaopectate 30 cubic centimeters orally twice daily as needed for diarrhea for length of stay
24. Tylenol ii tabs orally three times daily as needed for headache and/or temp above 101° F for length of stay
25. Motrin 600 mg orally every 6 hours as needed for muscle aches and pain for length of stay
26. Robitussin 10 ml orally every 4 hours as needed for cough for length of stay
27. Cepacol throat lozenges one orally every 4 hours as needed for sore throat for length of stay
28. Random Urine Drug Screen (as determined by nursing)
29. Complete the CIWA (for alcohol) if considering administration of PRN detox medication.

NOTE: This protocol may be adjusted at any time by the Medical Staff.

Routine Labs: ____ CBC   ____ Urinalysis
                 ____ SMAC   ____ Urine Drug Screen
                 ____ Urine Pregnancy Test   ____ Serum Pregnancy Test

Physician/APN Signature:_____Date: _____
Time:_____

ADULT ALCOHOL DETOXIFICATION PROTOCOL # 2
STANDING ORDERS

Patient Name: _____ **ID#:** _____

1. Admit to:
2. Regular Diet
3. Vital signs per policy
4. Administer 0.1cubic centimeters intradermally to left forearm Tuberculin Purified Protein Derivative; repeat in two weeks when applicable.
5. Multivitamins one tab orally daily for length of stay
6. Thiamine 100 milligrams orally twice daily for 5 Days, then
7. Thiamine 100 milligrams orally once daily thereafter for length of stay
8. Librium 75 milligrams orally as initial dose then
9. Librium 75 milligrams orally every 6 hours for 24 hours, then
10. Librium 50 milligrams orally every 6 hours for 24 hours, then
11. Librium 35 milligrams orally every 6 hours for 24 hours, then
12. Librium 25 milligrams orally every 6 hours for 24 hours, then
13. Librium 10 milligrams orally every 6 hours for 24 hours, then discontinue
14. Librium 25 milligrams orally every 4 hours as needed based on signs and symptoms of withdrawal for 5 days, then discontinue
15. Levsin 0.125 milligrams sublingually every 6 hours as needed for abdominal pain for 5 days

16. Vistaril 50 milligrams orally every 4 hours as needed for anxiety or agitation for length of stay
17. 48 hours after discontinuation of the detoxification protocol Campral 333 milligrams, (2 tablets) will be initiated orally three times per day
18. 48 hours after discontinuation of the detoxification protocol give Naltrexone 25 milligrams orally at bed time x 3 days then increase Naltrexone to 50 milligram once orally at bed time thereafter
19. Vivitrol 380 milligrams intramuscular to the gluteal region once monthly if patient fails Naltrexone oral challenge or if patient's liver enzymes are elevated. Notify medical staff to discuss Vivitrol therapy with the patient prior to initiation and also for written prescription.
20. Trazadone 50 milligrams orally at bed time as needed for insomnia for length of stay
21. May repeat Trazadone 50 milligrams orally 1 additional dose 2 hours after the first dose if the first dose is not effective as needed for insomnia for length of stay
22. Milk of Magnesia 30 cubic centimeters orally twice daily as needed for constipation for length of stay
23. Maalox 30 cubic centimeters orally twice daily as needed for indigestion for length of stay
24. Kaopectate 30 cubic centimeters orally twice daily as needed for diarrhea for length of stay
25. Tylenol ii tabs orally three times a day as needed for headache or temp above 101° F for length of stay
26. Motrin 600 milligrams orally every 6 hours as needed for muscle aches or pain for length of stay
27. Robitussin 10 milliliters orally every 4 hours as needed for cough for length of stay
28. Cepacol throat lozenges one orally every 4 hours as needed for sore throat for length of stay
29. Random Urine Drug Screen (as determined by nursing)
30. Complete the CIWA (for alcohol) if considering administration of PRN detox medication

NOTE: This protocol may be adjusted at any time by the Medical Staff.

Routine Labs: ____ CBC   ____Urinalysis
              ____ SMAC   ____Urine Drug Screen
              ____ Urine Pregnancy Test   ____Serum Pregnancy Test

Physician/APN Signature: _____Date: _____
Time: _____

ADULT ALCOHOL DETOXIFICATION PROTOCOL # 3
STANDING ORDERS

Patient Name: _____ **ID#:** _____

1. Admit to:
2. Regular Diet
3. Vital signs per policy
4. Administer 0.1cubic centimeters intradermally to left forearm Tuberculin Purified Protein Derivative; repeat in two weeks when applicable.

5. Multivitamins one tab orally daily for length of stay
6. Thiamine 100 milligrams orally twice daily for 5 days, then
7. Thiamine 100 milligrams orally once daily thereafter for length of stay
8. Librium 75 milligrams orally as initial dose then
9. Librium 75 milligrams orally every 6 hours for 24 hours, then
10. Librium 50 milligrams orally every 6 hours for 24 hours, then
11. Librium 35 milligrams orally every 6 hours for 24 hours, then
12. Librium 25 milligrams orally every 6 hours for 24 hours, then
13. Librium 10 milligrams orally every 6 hours for 24 hours, then discontinue
14. Librium 25 milligrams orally every 4 hours as needed based on signs and symptoms of withdrawal for 5 days, then discontinue
15. Levsin 0.125 milligrams sublingually every 6 hours as needed for abdominal cramps for 5 days
16. Vistaril 50 milligrams orally every 4 hours as needed for anxiety or agitation for length of stay
17. 48 hours after discontinuation of the detoxification protocol Campral 333 milligrams, (2 tablets) will be initiated orally three times per day
18. 48 hours after discontinuation of the detoxification protocol give Naltrexone 25 milligrams orally at bed time x 3 days then increase Naltrexone to 50 milligram once orally at bed time thereafter
19. Vivitrol 380 milligrams intramuscular to the gluteal region once monthly if patient fails Naltrexone oral challenge or if patient's liver enzymes are elevated. Notify medical staff to discuss Vivitrol therapy with the patient prior to initiation and also for written prescription.
20. Trazadone 50 milligrams orally at bed time as needed for insomnia for length of stay
21. May repeat Trazadone 50 milligrams orally 1 additional dose 2 hours after the first dose if the first dose is not effective as needed for insomnia for length of stay
22. Clonidine 0.2 milligrams orally now, then
23. Clonidine 0.1 milligrams orally every 6 hours for 24 hours, then
24. Clonidine 0.1 milligrams orally every 8 hours for 24 hours, then
25. Clonidine 0.1 milligrams orally every 12 hours for 24 hours, then discontinue
26. Hold Clonidine if systolic blood pressure is less than100 and/or heart rate is less than 50
27. Tegretol 200 milligrams orally twice daily for length of stay
28. Serum Tegretol Level in 5 days
29. Milk of Magnesia 30 cubic centimeters orally twice daily as needed for constipation for length of stay
30. Kaopectate 30 cubic centimeters orally twice daily as needed for diarrhea for length of stay
31. Tylenol ii tabs orally three times a day as needed for headache or temp above 101° F for length of stay
32. Motrin 600 milligrams orally every 6 hours as needed for muscle aches or pain for length of stay
33. Robitussin 10 milliliters orally every 4 hours as needed for cough for length of stay
34. Cepacol throat lozenges one orally every 4 hours as needed for sore throat for length of stay
35. Random Urine Drug Screen (as determined by nursing)
36. Complete the CIWA (for alcohol) if considering administration of PRN detox medication

NOTE: This protocol may be adjusted at any time by the Medical Staff.

Routine Labs: ____ CBC ____ SMAC ____Urinalysis ____Serum Pregnancy Test
____ Urine Pregnancy Test ____Urine Drug Screen

Physician/APN Signature: _____ Date: _____
Time: _____

ADULT OPIATE DETOXIFICATION PROTOCOL # 1
STANDING ORDERS

Patient Name: _____ **ID#:** _____

1. Admit to:
2. Regular Diet
3. Vital signs per policy
4. Administer 0.1cubic centimeters intradermally to left forearm Tuberculin Purified Protein Derivative; repeat in two weeks when applicable.
5. Multivitamins one tab orally daily for length of stay
6. Thiamine 100 milligrams orally once daily for length of stay
7. Phenobarbital 120 milligrams orally for 1 dose as needed and may repeat dose once as needed within a 24 hour time period
8. Phenobarbital 75 milligrams orally every 6 hours for 24 hours, then
9. Phenobarbital 60 milligrams orally every 6 hours for 24 hours, then
10. Phenobarbital 45 milligrams orally every 6 hours for 24 hours, then
11. Phenobarbital 30 milligrams orally every 6 hours for 24 hours, then
12. Phenobarbital 15 milligrams orally every 6 hours for 24 hours, then discontinue
13. Clonidine 0.1 milligrams orally every 6 hours for 48 hours, then
14. Clonidine 0.1 milligrams orally every 8 hours for 24 hours, then
15. Clonidine 0.1 milligrams orally every 12 hours for 24 hours, then discontinue
16. Hold Clonidine if systolic blood pressure is less than 100 mmHg. or heart rate is less than 50
17. Levsin 0.125 milligrams sublingually every 6 hours as needed for abdominal cramps for 5 days
18. Vistaril 50 milligrams orally every 4 hours as needed for anxiety or agitation for length of stay
19. Trazadone 50 milligrams orally at bed time as needed for insomnia for length of stay
20. May repeat Trazadone 50 milligrams orally 1 additional dose 2 hours after the first dose if the first dose is not effective as needed for insomnia for length of stay
21. Robaxin 1500 milligrams orally 3 times a day for 5 days
22. Flexeril 10 milligrams orally at bedtime for 5 days
23. Milk of Magnesia 30 cubic centimeters orally twice daily as needed for constipation for length of stay
24. Maalox 30 cubic centimeters orally twice daily as needed for indigestion for length of stay
25. Kaopectate 30 cubic centimeters orally twice daily as needed for diarrhea for length of stay
26. Tylenol ii tabs orally three times a day as needed for headache or temp above 101° F for length of stay

27. Motrin 600 milligrams orally every 6 hours as needed for muscle aches or pain for length of stay
28. Robitussin 10 milliliters orally every Q 4 hours as needed for cough for length of stay
29. Cepacol throat lozenges one orally every 4 hours as needed for sore throat for length of stay
30. Random Urine Drug Screen (as determined by nursing)
31. Complete the COWS (for opiates) if considering administration of PRN detox medication
32. Naltrexone 25 milligrams orally once daily at bedtime for 3 days, the increase Naltrexone to 50 milligrams orally once daily thereafter for length of stay.
33. Do not administer initial dose of Naltrexone until patient has been off all opioids for a 10 day time period

NOTE: This protocol may be adjusted at any time by the Medical Staff.

Routine Labs: ___ CBC   ___ Urinalysis
               ___ SMAC   ___ Urine Drug Screen
               ___ Urine Pregnancy test   ___ Serum Pregnancy test

Physician/APN Signature: _____ Date: _____
Time: _____

ADULT OPIATE DETOXIFICATION PROTOCOL # 2
STANDING ORDERS

Patient Name: _____ ID#: _____

1. Admit to:
2. Regular Diet
3. Vital signs per policy
4. Administer 0.1 cubic centimeters intradermally to left forearm Tuberculin Purified Protein Derivative; repeat in two weeks when applicable.
5. Multivitamins one tab orally daily for length of stay
6. Thiamine 100 milligrams orally once daily for length of stay
7. Phenobarbital 120 milligrams orally for 1 dose as needed and may repeat dose for 1 as needed within a 24 hour time period
8. Phenobarbital 60 milligrams orally every 6 hours for 24 hours, then
9. Phenobarbital 45 milligrams orally every 6 hours for 24 hours, then
10. Phenobarbital 30 milligrams orally every 6 hours for 24 hours, then
11. Phenobarbital 15 milligrams orally every 6 hours for 24 hours, then discontinue
12. Phenobarbital 30 milligrams orally every 6 hours as needed based on the signs and symptoms of withdrawal for 5 days
13. Clonidine 0.1 milligrams orally every 6 hours for 48 hours, then
14. Clonidine 0.1 milligrams orally every 8 hours for 24 hours, then
15. Clonidine 0.1 milligrams orally every 12 hours for 24 hours, then discontinue
16. Hold Clonidine if systolic blood pressure is less than 100 mm Hg. or heart rate is less than 50

17. Levsin 0.125 milligrams sublingually every 6 hours as needed abdominal cramps for 5 days
18. Vistaril 50 milligrams orally every 4 hours as needed for anxiety or agitation for length of stay
19. Robaxin 1500 milligrams orally 3 times a day for 5 days
20. Flexeril 10 milligrams orally at bedtime for 5 days
21. Trazadone 50 milligrams orally at bed time as needed for insomnia for length of stay
22. May repeat Trazadone 50 milligrams orally 1 additional dose 2 hours after the first dose if the first dose is not effective as needed for insomnia for length of stay
23. Milk of Magnesia 30 cubic centimeters orally twice daily as needed for constipation for length of stay
24. Maalox 30 cubic centimeters orally twice daily as needed for indigestion for length of stay
25. Kaopectate 30 cubic centimeters orally twice daily as needed for diarrhea for length of stay
26. Tylenol ii tabs orally three times a day as needed for headache or temp above 101° F for length of stay
27. Motrin 600 milligrams orally every 6 hours as needed for muscle aches or pain for length of stay
28. Robitussin 10 milliliters orally every 4 as needed for cough for length of stay
29. Cepacol throat lozenges one orally every 4 hours as needed for sore throat for length of stay
30. Random Urine Drug Screen (as determined by nursing)
31. Complete the COWS (for opiates) if considering administration of PRN detox medication
32. Naltrexone 25 milligrams orally once daily at bedtime for 3 days, the increase Naltrexone to 50 milligrams orally once daily thereafter for length of stay.
33. Do not administer initial dose of Naltrexone until patient has been off all opioids for a 10 day time period.

NOTE: This protocol may be adjusted at any time by the Medical Staff.

Routine Labs: ___ CBC   ___ Urinalysis
               ___ SMAC   ___ Urine Drug Screen
               ___ Urine Pregnancy test   ___ Serum Pregnancy test

Physician/APNSignature: _____ Date: _____
Time: _____

ADULT OPIATE DETOXIFICATION PROTOCOL # 3
STANDING ORDERS

Patient Name: _____ **ID#:** _____

1. Admit to:
2. Regular Diet
3. Vital signs per policy
4. Administer 0.1 cubic centimeters intradermally to left forearm Tuberculin Purified Protein Derivative; repeat in two weeks when applicable.
5. Multivitamins one tab orally daily for length of stay

6. Thiamine 100 milligrams orally once daily for length of stay
7. Methadone 20 milligrams orally today
8. Reduce Methadone daily by 5 milligrams until dose is 0 milligrams. Begin order 12 hours after initial dose of Methadone.
9. Clonidine 0.1 milligrams orally every 6 hours for 24 hours, then reduce to
10. Clonidine 0.1 milligrams orally every 8 hours for 24 hours, then reduce to
11. Clonidine 0.1 milligrams orally every 12 hours for 24 hours, then discontinue
12. Hold Clonidine if systolic blood pressure is less than 100 millimeters Hg. or heart rate is less than 50
13. Librium 25 milligrams orally every 6 hours for 24 hours, then reduce to
14. Librium 25 milligrams orally every 8 hours for 24 hours, then reduce to
15. Librium 10 milligrams orally every 8 hours for 24 hours, then discontinue
16. Librium 25 milligrams orally every 6 hours as needed based on signs and symptoms of withdrawal for 5 days
17. Levsin 0.125 milligrams sublingually every 6 hours as needed abdominal cramps for 5 days
18. Vistaril 50 milligrams orally every 4 hours as needed for anxiety or agitation for length of stay
19. Robaxin 1500 milligrams orally 3 times a day for 5 days
20. Flexeril 10 milligrams orally at bedtime for 5 days
21. Trazadone 50 milligrams orally at bed time as needed for insomnia for length of stay
22. May repeat Trazadone 50 milligrams orally 1 additional dose 2 hours after the first dose if the first dose is not effective as needed for insomnia for length of stay
23. Milk of Magnesia 30 cubic centimeters orally twice daily as needed for constipation for length of stay
24. Maalox 30 cubic centimeters orally twice daily as needed for indigestion for length of stay
25. Kaopectate 30 cubic centimeters orally twice daily as needed for diarrhea for length of stay
26. Tylenol ii tabs orally three times a day as needed for headache or temp above 101° F for length of stay
27. Motrin 600 milligrams orally every 6 hours as needed for muscle aches or pain for length of stay
28. Robitussin 10 milliliters orally every 4 hours as needed for cough for length of stay
29. Cepacol throat lozenges one orally every 4 hours as needed for sore throat for length of stay
30. Random Urine Drug Screen (as determined by nursing)
31. Complete the COWS (for opiates) if considering administration of PRN detox medication
32. Naltrexone 25 milligrams orally once daily at bedtime for 3 days, the increase Naltrexone to 50 milligrams orally once daily thereafter for length of stay.
33. Do not administer initial dose of Naltrexone until patient has been off Methadone and all opioids for a 10 day time period.

NOTE: This protocol may be adjusted at any time by the Medical Staff.

Routine Labs: ___ CBC   ___ Urinalysis
              ___ SMAC   ___ Urine Drug Screen
              ___ Urine Pregnancy test ___ Serum Pregnancy test

Physician/APN Signature: _____ Date: _____
Time: _____

ADULT OPIATE DETOXIFICATION PROTOCOL # 4
STANDING ORDERS

Patient Name: _____ **ID#:** _____

1. Admit to:
2. Regular Diet
3. Vital signs per policy
4. Administer 0.1 cc intradermally to left forearm Tuberculin Purified Protein Derivative; repeat in two weeks when applicable.
5. Multivitamins one tab orally daily for length of stay
6. Thiamine 100 milligrams orally once daily for length of stay
7. Methadone 25 milligrams orally today
8. Reduce Methadone daily by 5 milligrams until dose is 0 milligrams. Begin order 12 hours after the initial dose of Methadone.
9. Clonidine 0.1 milligrams orally every 6 hours for 24 hours, then reduce to
10. Clonidine 0.1 milligrams orally every 8 hours for 24 hours, then reduce to
11. Clonidine 0.1 milligrams orally every 12 hours for 24 hours, then discontinue
12. Hold Clonidine if systolic blood pressure is less than 100 millimeters Hg. or heart rate is less than 50
13. Librium 25 milligrams orally every 6 hours for 24 hours, then reduce to
14. Librium 25 milligrams orally every 8 hours for 24 hours, then reduce to
15. Librium 10 milligrams orally every 8 hours for 24 hours, then discontinue
16. Librium 25 milligrams orally every 6 hours as needed based on signs and symptoms of withdrawal for 5 days
17. Levsin 0.125 milligrams sublingually every 6 hours as needed for abdominal cramps for 5 days
18. Vistaril 50 milligrams orally every 4 hours as needed for anxiety or agitation for length of stay
19. Robaxin 1500 milligrams orally 3 times a day for 5 days
20. Flexeril 10 milligrams orally at bedtime for 5 days
21. Trazadone 50 milligrams orally at bed time as needed for insomnia for length of stay
22. May repeat Trazadone 50 milligrams orally 1 additional dose 2 hours after the first dose if the first dose is not effective as needed for insomnia for length of stay
23. Milk of Magnesia 30 cubic centimeters orally twice daily as needed for constipation for length of stay
24. Maalox 30 cubic centimeters orally twice daily as needed for indigestion for length of stay
25. Kaopectate 30 cubic centimeters orally twice daily as needed for diarrhea for length of stay
26. Tylenol ii tabs orally three times a day as needed for headache or temp above 101° F for length of stay
27. Motrin 600 milligrams orally every 6 hours as needed for muscle aches or pain for length of stay
28. Robitussin 10 milliliters orally every 4 hours as needed for cough for length of stay
29. Cepacol throat lozenges one orally every 4 hours as needed/ for sore throat for length of stay
30. Random Urine Drug Screen (as determined by nursing)

31. Complete the COWS (for opiates) if considering administration of PRN detox medication
32. Naltrexone 25 milligrams orally once daily at bedtime for 3 days, the increase Naltrexone to 50 milligrams orally once daily thereafter for length of stay.
33. Do not administer initial dose of Naltrexone until patient has been off Methadone and all opioids for a 10 day time period.

NOTE: This protocol may be adjusted at any time by the Medical Staff.

Routine Labs: ___ CBC   ___ Urinalysis ___ Urine Drug Screen
              ___ SMAC   ___ Urine Pregnancy test ___ Serum Pregnancy test

Physician/APN Signature: _____ Date: _____
Time: _____

ADULT OPIATE DETOXIFICATION PROTOCOL # 5
STANDING ORDERS

Patient Name: _____ **ID#:** _____

1. Admit to:
2. Regular Diet
3. Vital signs per policy
4. Administer 0.1 cubic centimeters intradermally to left forearm Tuberculin Purified Protein Derivative; repeat in two weeks when applicable.
5. Multivitamins one tab orally daily for length of stay
6. Thiamine 100 milligrams orally once daily for length of stay
7. Methadone 30 milligrams orally today
8. Reduce Methadone daily by 5 milligrams until dose is 0 milligrams. Begin order 12 hours after initial dose of Methadone.
9. Librium 25 milligrams orally every 6 hours as needed for 5 days
10. Levsin 0.125 milligrams sublingually every 6 hours as needed abdominal cramps for 5 days
11. Vistaril 50 milligrams orally every 4 hours as needed for anxiety for length of stay
12. Robaxin 1500 milligrams orally 3 times a day for 5 days
13. Flexeril 10 milligrams orally at bedtime for 5 days
14. Trazadone 50 milligrams orally at bed time as needed for insomnia for length of stay
15. May repeat Trazadone 50 milligrams orally 1 additional dose 2 hours after the first dose if the first dose is not effective as needed for insomnia for length of stay
16. Milk of Magnesia 30 cubic centimeters orally twice daily as needed for constipation for length of stay
17. Maalox 30 cubic centimeters orally twice daily as needed for indigestion for length of stay
18. Kaopectate 30 cubic centimeters orally twice daily as needed for diarrhea for length of stay
19. Tylenol ii tabs orally three times a day as needed/headache or temp above 101° F for length of stay

20. Motrin 600 milligrams orally every 6 hours as needed for muscle aches or pain for length of stay
21. Robitussin 10 milliliters orally every 4 hours as needed for cough for length of stay
22. Cepacol throat Lozenges one orally every 4 hours as needed for sore throat for length of stay
23. Random Urine Drug Screen (as determined by nursing)
24. Complete the COWS (for opiates) if considering administration of PRN detox medication
25. Naltrexone 25 milligrams orally once daily at bedtime for 3 days, the increase Naltrexone to 50 milligrams orally once daily thereafter for length of stay.
26. Do not administer initial dose of Naltrexone until patient has been off Methadone and all opioids for a 10 day time period.

NOTE: This protocol may be adjusted at any time by the Medical Staff.

Routine Labs: ___ CBC   ___ Urinalysis
                 ___ SMAC   ___ Urine Drug Screen
                 ___ Urine Pregnancy test   ___ Serum Pregnancy test

Physician/APN Signature: _____ Date: _____
Time: _____

ADULT OPIATE DETOXIFICATION PROTOCOL # 6
STANDING ORDERS

Patient Name: _____ **ID#:** _____

1. Admit to:
2. Diet: _____
3. Vital signs per policy
4. Administer 0.1cubic centimeters intradermally to left forearm Tuberculin Purified Protein Derivative; repeat in two weeks when applicable.
5. Buprenorphine 0.3 milligrams base/milliliters, intramuscularly every 6 hrs for 24 hrs, then Buprenorphine 0.3 milligrams base/milliliters, intramuscularly every 8 hrs for 24 hrs, then
6. Suboxone 8 milligrams orally once daily for 24 hours, then
7. Suboxone 4 milligrams orally once daily for 24 hours, then discontinue
8. Multivitamins one tab orally daily for length of stay
9. Vistaril 50 milligrams orally every 6 hours as needed for anxiety or agitation for length of stay
10. Robaxin 1500 milligrams orally 3 times a day for 5 days
11. Flexeril 10 milligrams orally at bedtime for 5 days
12. Trazadone 50 milligrams orally at bed time as needed for insomnia for length of stay
13. May repeat Trazadone 50 milligrams orally 1 additional dose 2 hours after the first dose if the first dose is not effective as needed for insomnia for length of stay
14. Milk of Magnesia 30 cubic centimeters orally twice daily as needed for constipation for length of stay

15. Maalox 30 cubic centimeters orally twice daily as needed for indigestion for length of stay
16. Kaopectate 30 cubic centimeters orally twice daily as needed for diarrhea for length of stay
17. Tylenol ii tabs orally three times a day as needed/headache or temp above 101° F for length of stay
18. Motrin 600 milligrams orally every 6 hours as needed for muscle aches or pain for length of stay
19. Robitussin 10 milliliters orally every 4 hours as needed for cough for length of stay
20. Cepacol throat Lozenges one orally every 4 hours as needed for sore throat for length of stay
21. Random Urine Drug Screen (as determined by nursing)
22. Complete the COWS (for opiates) if considering administration of PRN detox medication

NOTE: This protocol may be adjusted at any time by the Medical Staff.

Routine Labs: ___ CBC   ___ Urinalysis
              ___ SMAC   ___ Urine Drug Screen
              ___ Urine Pregnancy test   ___ Serum Pregnancy test

Physician/APN Signature: _____ Date: _____
Time: _____

ADULT BENZODIAZEPINE DETOXIFICATION PROTOCOL # 1
STANDING ORDERS

Patient Name: _____ **ID#:** _____

1. Admit to:
2. Regular Diet
3. Vital signs per policy
4. Administer 0.1cubic centimeters intradermally to left forearm Tuberculin Purified Protein Derivative; repeat in two weeks when applicable.
5. Multivitamins one tab orally daily for length of stay
6. Thiamine 100 milligrams orally once daily for length of stay
7. Phenobarbital 120 milligrams orally for 1 dose as needed and may repeat dose once as needed within a 24 hour time period
8. Phenobarbital 75 milligrams orally every 6 hours for 24 hours, then
9. Phenobarbital 60 milligrams orally every 6 hours for 24 hours, then
10. Phenobarbital 45 milligrams orally every 6 hours for 24 hours, then
11. Phenobarbital 30 milligrams orally every 6 hours for 24 hours, then
12. Phenobarbital 15 milligrams orally every 6 hours for 24 hours, then discontinue
13. Phenobarbital 30 milligrams orally every 6 hours as needed based on signs and symptoms
14. Clonidine 0.1 milligrams orally every 6 hours for 48 hours, then
15. Clonidine 0.1 milligrams orally every 8 hours for 24 hours, then
16. Clonidine 0.1 milligrams orally every 12 hours for 24 hours, then discontinue
17. Hold Clonidine if systolic blood pressure is less 100 and/or heart rate is less than 50

18. Levsin 0.125 milligrams sublingually every 6 hours as needed for abdominal cramps for 5 days
19. Vistaril 50 milligrams orally every 4 hours as needed for anxiety or agitation for length of stay
20. Tegretol 200 milligrams orally twice daily for length of stay
21. Serum Tegretol Level in 5 days
22. Seizure Precautions
23. Trazadone 50 milligrams orally at bed time as needed for insomnia for length of stay
24. May repeat Trazadone 50 milligrams orally 1 additional dose 2 hours after the first dose if the first dose is not effective as needed for insomnia for length of stay
25. Milk of Magnesia 30 cubic centimeters orally twice daily as needed for constipation for length of stay
26. Maalox 30 cubic centimeters orally twice daily as needed for indigestion for length of stay
27. Kaopectate 30 cubic centimeters orally twice daily as needed for diarrhea for length of stay
28. Tylenol ii tabs orally three times a day as needed for headache or temp above 101° F for length of stay
29. Motrin 600 milligrams orally every 6 hours as needed for muscle aches or pain for length of stay
30. Robitussin 10 milliliters orally every 4 hours as needed for cough for length of stay
31. Cepacol throat lozenges one orally every 4 hours as needed for sore throat for length of stay
32. Random Urine Drug Screen (as determined by nursing)

NOTE: This protocol may be adjusted at any time by the Medical Staff.

Routine Labs: ___ CBC   ___ Urinalysis
              ___ SMAC   ___ Urine Drug Screen
              ___ Urine Pregnancy test   ___ Serum Pregnancy test

Physician/APN Signature: _____ Date: _____
Time: _____

REFERENCES

1. Ott PJ, Tarter RE, Ammerman RT. Sourcebook on substance abuse: etiology, epidemiology, assessment and treatment. Boston (MA): Allyn and Bacon; 1999.
2. Lejoyeux M, Solomon J, Ades J. Benzodiazepine treatment for alcohol-dependent patients. Alcohol Alcohol 1998;33(6):563–75.
3. Phillips S, Haycock C, Boyle D. Development of an alcohol withdrawal protocol: CNS collaborative exemplar. Clin Nurse Spec 2006;20(4):190–8.
4. Nimmerrichter AA, Walter H, Gutierrez-Lobos KE, et al. Double-blind controlled trial of hydroxybutyrate and clomethiazole in the treatment of alcohol withdrawal. Alcohol Alcohol 2002;37(1):67–73.
5. Streeter C, Whelan G. Naltrexone, a relapse prevention maintenance treatment of alcohol dependence: a meta-analysis of randomized control trials. Alcohol Alcohol 2001;36(6):544–52.
6. Brown B. Use of alcohol by addict and non-addict populations. Am J Psychiatry 1973;130:599–601.

7. Liebson I, Bigelow G, Flamer R. Alcoholism among methadone patients: a specific treatment method. Am J Psychiatry 1973;130:483–5.
8. El-Bassel N, Shilling RF, Turnbull JE, et al. Correlates of alcohol use among methadone patients. Alcohol Clin Exp Res 1993;17:681–6.
9. Caputo F, Addolorato G, Domenicali M, et al. Short-term methadone administration reduces alcohol consumption in non-alcoholic heroin addicts. Alcohol Alcohol 2002;37(2):164–8.
10. Fiellin DA, Rosenheck RA, Kosten TR. Office-based treatment of opioid dependence: reaching new patient populations. Am J Psychiatry 2001;158(8):1200–4.
11. Carroll KM, Ball SA, Nich C, et al. Targeting behavioral therapies to enhance naltrexone treatment of opioid dependence. Arch Gen Psychiatry 2001;58: 755–61.

Maintaining Sobriety and Recovery

William J. Lorman, PhD, MSN, PMHNP-BC, CARN-AP[a,b],*

KEYWORDS

- Addiction treatment • Abstinence • Sobriety • Recovery • Relapse
- Substance use disorder

KEY POINTS

- Addiction is a chronic, progressive disease, and if not treated, it is fatal.
- Maintaining sobriety means only that the person is not using drugs or alcohol and does not mean that the person has made any other changes in his or her life.
- Recovery is a process of change through which individuals improve their health and wellness, live a self-directed life, and strive to reach their full potential.

INTRODUCTION

In general parlance, the word recovery, as it relates to health, is defined by the Merriam–Webster Dictionary[1] as "the process of combating a disorder or problem." Over the years, people working with patients being treated for a substance use disorder have used this or a variant of this definition. But ask for a definition, and one will probably get as many definitions as the number of people asked. For the most part, one tends to emphasize the "combating a disorder or problem" as the goal, and forget or minimize the "process" part of the definition. Those in recovery know what it means to them, but it is not clear to the public.[2] A common cause of confusion for many clinicians is the terminology and definitions of the Diagnostic and Statistical Manual of Mental Disorders (Fourth Edition, Text Revision) (DSM-IV-TR)[3] course specifiers for substance dependence. The DSM-IV-TR uses the term remission, and many clinicians use this interchangeably for recovery. There are 4 remission specifiers used, and all relate in 1 way or another to the patient meeting at least 1 dependence criterion (partial remission) or none (full remission), and for how long a period, such as from 1 month up to a year (early remission) or longer than a year (sustained remission). But being in recovery is much more than being in remission from the disease. In general, those pursuing recovery want improved function and a satisfying quality of life.[4]

The author has nothing to disclose.
[a] Livengrin Foundation, Inc, Bensalem, PA, USA; [b] Drexel University College of Nursing & Health Professions, Philadelphia, PA, USA
* Corresponding author. Livengrin Foundation, Inc, 4833 Hulmeville Road, Bensalem, PA 19020.
E-mail address: wlorman@livengrin.org

Over the years, the Substance Abuse and Mental Health Services Administration (SAMHSA) has published various definitions of recovery, but in August, 2011, it developed a newly revised and updated definition and then published it[5] as follows:

"A process of change through which individuals improve their health and wellness, live a self-directed life, and strive to reach their full potential."

This definition is quite complete. It is user-friendly and can be used as a template for a treatment outcomes plan for any patient suffering from the disease of addiction. It also clarifies that recovery is a process rather than an endpoint, in itself a veritable myth breaker. Further, the definition is consistent with the World Health Organization's conceptualization of health as "a state of complete physical, mental and social well-being, not merely the absence of disease."[6] Also, as part of this undertaking, SAMHSA[5] delineated 4 major dimensions of health, home, purpose, and community that should be used to support an addicted person's life in recovery. These are further explained in **Box 1**. Of course the Alcoholics Anonymous Organization, in its eponymous text[7] (also referred to as "The Big Book") has espoused a similar explanation of recovery along with adjunctive behavioral outcomes. It is unfortunate that there are many clinicians—those without a history of an addictive disorder and no understanding of recovery—who are not intimately familiar with the contents of the "Big Book" which, in itself, is an excellent primer on the treatment of addiction (alcoholism) and the means to sustained recovery.

GETTING TO SOBRIETY

Before one can speak to a program for sustained recovery, one must first address the process of addiction itself and then the movement toward sobriety. The predominant and most accepted model explaining addiction is the disease model. This model, which is based on a genetic predisposition for the disease, is accepted by both the American Psychiatric Association[3] and Alcoholics Anonymous.[7] From a behavioral/psychiatric perspective, observable symptoms include substance use (alcohol or other drug), identifiable behaviors (the consequences and inappropriate behaviors attributed to the addicted person during periods of intoxication, withdrawal, being

---

Box 1
The 4 major dimensions that support a life in recovery

Health

Overcoming or managing one's disease(s) as well as living in a physically and emotionally healthy way

Home

A stable and safe place to live

Purpose

Meaningful daily activities, such as a job, school, volunteerism, family caretaking, or creative endeavors, and the independence, income, and resources to participate in society

Community

Relationships and social networks that provide support, friendship, love, and hope

From Substance Abuse and Mental Health Services Administration. SAMHSA news release. 2012. Available at: http://blog.samhsa.gov/2012/03/23/defintion-of-recovery-updated/. Accessed October 24, 2012.

distracted at the thoughts of getting and using the substance, and a decrease in social functioning) which are captured very well in the DSM-IV-TR's criterion number 6 found in the criteria set for substance dependence and express the increasing manifestation of important social, occupational, or other activities given up or reduced because of the substance use.[3]

Addiction is also categorized as chronic, progressive and, if not treated, fatal. This reflects the medical model of any chronic disease and places addiction on the same (biologic) level as hypertension, diabetes, and chronic obstructive pulmonary disease (COPD). Being a chronic condition, addiction may not have a complete or permanent solution. That is, there is no cure, only treatment to better manage the condition.[8] According to the psychoanalytic model, addiction serves some purpose, and once that purpose is determined as applied to the individual, then insight into the disease can occur.[9] Alcoholics Anonymous, for decades, has described the cues or relapse triggers of "people, places and things." It is now known, through the study of neurobiology, that 1 role of the thalamus is to act as a relay center for all sensory input, and it is regulated by the immediate needs of the individual.[10] For example, when an alcohol-naïve person (one who does not have an alcohol addiction) walks into a bar, he or she is alerted to the strongest sensory stimuli in the room, such as flashing lights, loud noises, and the furniture in the room. A person who has an alcohol addiction will first notice the smell of alcoholic beverages and the bottles of alcohol on the shelves. This demonstrates nicely how "people, places and things" can lead to relapse, because they become the center of addiction-related history and therefore are imprinted in the thalamic pathways leading to the action of using alcohol again.

Treatment is both content- and process-oriented. The drugs and alcohol themselves are the content, and sobriety refers to the removal of content, in other words, abstinence from drug and alcohol use. Process refers to the behaviors that the addicted person has incorporated as part of his or her activities of daily living that are dysfunctional, inappropriate, and often pathologic. SAMHSA[11] has identified early predictors of success in maintaining sobriety such as having housing, maintaining a productive job, having no legal involvement, maintaining a support network such as 12-step meeting attendance, and maintaining abstinence. Problems related to these issues are associated with poor retention in treatment, poor treatment outcomes, and a higher probability of relapse.[12] There has been much controversy over the past decade about the role of abstinence versus harm reduction, controlled use of substances in decreasing quantities than previously used. However, most treatment centers, even today, encourage embracing abstinence as a recovery goal. Most failed attempts to remain sober have been shown to be a result of moderation ("controlled use"), and abstinence has proven to be more successful.[13] Abstinence, especially sustained abstinence, has itself been associated with quality of life improvements.[14]

DELIVERY OF SERVICES

A basic assumption in delivery of services is that there be access to care. Unfortunately, there are many areas across the United States where specialized care for persons with substance use disorders is not available. Additionally, a person may be limited to a few select providers who are in the person's managed care network, and even though there may be a facility nearby, the person is directed to a provider who may be 50 to 100 miles away. Another major obstacle in accessing treatment is that many health care insurance products no longer provide a substance abuse benefit.[15] As a result of the many impediments in accessing care, only 9% of those who need treatment actually receive it. It is hoped that health care reform may alleviate this problem. Providing comprehensive, integrated services is another important aspect of care. When a patient presents for treatment, it is extremely rare that he or she has the singular problem of substance misuse. In fact, most have co-occurring psychiatric and medical problems in addition to many other psychosocial problems including job jeopardy, family discord, financial issues, or legal problems.[16] Treatment, if it be successful, must address all these issues, most of which are triggers for relapse. Finally, treatment must ensure continuity of care. Another unfortunate reality is that many treatment facilities and providers discharge the patient to home (or worse, to the street) without ensuring the patient has adequate ego strength and support services to remain sober and begin working toward sustained recovery.

GETTING TO RECOVERY

The clinician, in preparing to help the person begin the process of recovery, must employ a recovery perspective. Addressing only the substance use is likely to lead to poor prognostic outcomes, including relapse, unless other issues and consequences related to the substance use are also addressed.[17] Recovery is a long-term process of internal change, and these changes proceed through various stages. Treatment interventions should be specific to the tasks and challenges faced at each stage of the process. A multiproblem viewpoint should also be adopted, since, as previously stated, patients have an array of mental health, medical, substance abuse, family, and social problems; treatment should address the immediate and long-term needs early in treatment, including building a supportive network. Because patients can have ongoing cognitive and functional impairments for up to 6 months (sometimes longer) after the last drug/alcohol use as a result of the brain recalibrating itself, use relatively short, highly structured treatment sessions that are focused on practical life problems. Also, begin to establish support systems to help maintain and extend treatment effectiveness. This system includes self-help groups, family support, and the patient's faith community. The Substance Abuse and Mental Health Services Administration has developed "Guiding Principles of Recovery" to help the clinician understand the complex nature of the recovery process. These principles are listed in **Table 1**.

FACTORS ASSOCIATED WITH POOR OUTCOME

Just as one should build upon the patient's strengths, one should also identify and neutralize issues that increase the risk for relapse. The first issue to determine and address is acceptance of illness. If the patient does not accept that there is a problem, then he or she will have no desire to change. Here, understanding the stages of change and using motivational interviewing skills will help the clinician better deal with the patient and help the patient remain engaged in treatment.[18] If the severity of the substance use disorder is determined to be high, the patient will be more engrained in his or her dysfunctional life, and brain chemistry may be irreversibly altered. This requires a complete assessment and the development of a treatment plan that identifies the significant issues as discussed previously.

Mee-Lee[19] has identified that no matter how intense the treatment experience or how high the quality of services provided, unless the patient has an adequate social or family support system, relapse becomes almost a certainty. Therefore, the clinician should, from the beginning of treatment, help the patient identify, build, and maintain his or her supports who will be available continually as necessary to help the patient remain sober and solidify efforts toward recovery. This is especially necessary in

Table 1	
Guiding principles of recovery	
Recovery emerges from hope	Believing that recovery is real provides the message of a better future, that people can overcome the obstacles that confront them.
Recovery is person-driven	Self-efficacy is the foundation for recovery as individuals define their own life goals.
Recovery occurs via many pathways	Individuals are unique with distinct needs, strengths, and backgrounds that affect their pathway to recovery. Abstinence is the safest approach.
Recovery is holistic	Recovery encompasses an individual's whole life. The array of services and supports available should be integrated and coordinated.
Recovery is supported by peers and allies	Mutual support, including the sharing of experiential knowledge and skills, plays an invaluable role in recovery.
Recovery is supported through relationships and social networks	An important factor is the presence and involvement of people who believe in the person's ability to recover.
Recovery is culturally based and influenced	Culture, including values, traditions, and beliefs, is crucial in determining a person's journey to recovery.
Recovery is supported by addressing trauma	Services and supports should be trauma-informed to foster safety and trust.
Recovery involves individual, family, and community strengths and responsibility	All these serve as a foundation for recovery.
Recovery is based on respect	Acceptance and appreciation for people affected by substance use and other problems are crucial in achieving recovery.

Adapted from SAMHSA's guiding principles of recovery. 2011. Available at: http://www.samhsa.gov/newsroom/advisories/1112223420.aspx. Accessed November 21, 2012.

the presence of poor coping skills. Most of these patients lack healthy coping skills to help them deal with day-to-day stressors.

RELAPSE RISK FACTORS

Recovery is a complex process, and the patient, along with his or her supports, must be ever alert to the relapse risk factors that must constantly be identified, then maneuvered around or resolved. Affective variables, such as the various mood states (eg, anger, anxiety, boredom, depression, emptiness, and loneliness), are regularly experienced by newly sober individuals. And it is not necessarily the mood in and of itself, but the patient's inability to cope with it that contributes to relapse. Poor coping skills, inability to manage stress, and inadequate problem-solving skills increase risk for relapse unless they are addressed early in treatment.

Environmental variables, "places" as identified by Alcoholics Anonymous, include availability of substances, social pressures to engage in substance use or stop taking prescribed medications, and homelessness; these are stressors that the patient may not always be able to avoid. Discussing how these things might affect the patient and preparing him or her to deal with them with proper supports is most important. There is also that area referred to as the spiritual variables that increase risk for relapse. These include excessive guilt and shame, lack of meaning or purpose in life, and lack of a belief in the need for help and support from others or a higher power. Both clinician and patient need to address these often minimized risks.

Issues within the treatment experience itself may create risk factors and should be identified and resolved in an aggressive manner. These include poor adherence to treatment, insufficient or wrong types of medications prescribed, inappropriate advice or interventions, and failure to respond to early warning signs of relapse. When assessing treatment failures in retrospect, many of these risk factors were present but either not properly identified or not addressed aggressively.

CLINICAL INTERVENTIONS TO REDUCE RELAPSE RISK

Unfortunately, some patients have so many relapse risk factors that addressing each is impossible. Remember, by the time the patient presents for treatment, there often has been a global deterioration in functionality so that coping mechanisms, support systems, ego strength, and impulse control are practically nonexistent. Some of the more generalized approaches should be considered, such as social skills training, cognitive reframing, assertiveness training, and stress management. Additionally, ability by both the patient and the clinician to identify and manage relapse warning signs should be a primary goal. Such signs usually appear as changes in the patient's attitudes, emotions, thoughts, and feelings. When the patient begins to miss sessions, participates less and less in 12-step programs, and shows symptoms of co-occurring disorders (usually because he or she has stopped taking medications), these are referred to as treatment destructive resistances that require immediate attention. The risk of relapse has increased significantly, and therefore relapse is probably imminent, if it has not already occurred.

Difficulty managing negative emotional states is considered the most common relapse precipitant, and helping the patient manage these emotions is imperative. And as previously mentioned, patients who have supportive family and social support systems are more likely to experience a better recovery than those who do not. Helping the patient resist social pressures is another task for the clinician. Have the patient discuss high-risk situations in which social pressure will be strong or in which he or she feels especially vulnerable. Develop and practice refusal skills with the patient and also challenge faulty beliefs such as "I can't have fun unless I use alcohol or drugs with these people; they won't accept me." Finally, teach the patient to identify cues or precipitants that lead to cravings or desires to use substances. This can be accomplished by using an inventory or symptom review checklist, building structure into daily life, and also coping with emergency situations.

MEDICATION-ASSISTED RECOVERY

There is much debate among 12-step groups, professional organizations, and individual clinicians as to whether medication-assisted abstinence and recovery is helpful or even whether the person is in a state of sobriety/recovery when taking psychoactive substances, even when prescribed. Most providers believe that medication-assisted treatment is not only helpful but is recognized as an instrument for sustained recovery. In order to appease many of the detractors, the author and colleagues have expanded the term abstinent to mean either medication-free abstinence or medication-assisted abstinence.

The issue as it stands is really not so much that medications such as methadone, buprenorphine, and modafinil are prescribed, but rather how the patient is managed during the prescription period. It is unfortunate that so often medication management is really only prescription writing with very little ongoing assessment of the patient regarding therapeutic effects, side effects, and most importantly, evaluating the success of the recovery process and also including the support systems involved with the patient's care.

SUMMARY

Recovery is a complex process that requires ongoing attention by the patient. Helping the patient begin the process is a task that the clinician assumes starting with the process of detoxification, where withdrawal symptoms are managed, through abstinence and sustained sobriety and finally preparing for recovery. With time, the patient becomes more able to maintain recovery by making changes in his or her life, improving health and becoming productive and successful in their roles whatever they may be: parent, employee, spouse, student.

The nurse is in a unique position to work with this population, because nurses view the patient holistically and consider the full spectrum of bio-psycho-socio-spiritual treatment and are fully able to implement various interventions. Nurses, to be most successful in treating persons with an addictive disorder, must commit to further continuing education to obtain the necessary knowledge, skills, and experience, along with implementing evidence-based practices and ultimately conducting the necessary research to help the nursing profession and the addiction treatment profession find better solutions and develop better outcomes for this population.

It is unfortunate that there are few studies examining the impact of clinician interventions on sustained recovery. And the studies themselves have produced inconsistent results. Some have found positive outcomes as assessed by the Addiction Severity Index,[20,21] and some have found no evidence of an effect.[22]

REFERENCES

1. Meriam-Webster's collegiate dictionary. 11th edition. Springfield (MA): Merriam-Webster, Inc; 2004.
2. Laudet A. What does recovery mean to you? Lessons from the recovery experience for research and practice. J Subst Abuse Treat 2007;33:243–56.
3. Diagnostic and statistical manual of mental disorders. 4th edition. Washington, DC: American Psychiatric Association; 2000. Text Revision (DSM-IV-TR).
4. Ware NC, Hopper K, Tugenber T, et al. Connectedness and citizenship: redefining social integration. Psychiatr Serv 2007;58:27–38.
5. Substance Abuse and Mental Health Services Administration. SAMHSA news release. 2012. Available at: http://blog.samhsa.gov/2012/03/23/defintion-of-recovery-updated/. Accessed November 20, 2012.
6. World Health Organization. Basic documents. 35th edition. Geneva (Switzerland): WHO; 1985.
7. Alcoholics anonymous. 4th edition. New York: Alcoholics Anonymous World Services, Inc; 2001.
8. Moos R, Moos B. Sixteen-year differential changes and stable remission among treated and untreated individuals with alcohol use disorders. Drug Alcohol Depend 2005;80:337–47.
9. Freud S. The standard edition of the complete psychological works of Sigmund Freud. New York: W.W.Norton & Co; 1959.

10. Charney D, Nestler E. Neurobiology of mental illness. 2nd edition. New York: Oxford University Press; 2004.
11. Substance Abuse and Mental Health Services Administration. Guiding principles and elements of recovery-oriented systems of care: what do we know from the research? 2009. Available at: http://partnersforrecovery.samhsa.gov/docs/Guiding_Principles_Whitepaper.pdf. Accessed November 20, 2012.
12. Simpson DD, Joe GW, Fletcher BW, et al. A national evaluation of treatment outcomes for cocaine dependence. Arch Gen Psychiatry 1999;56:507–14.
13. Maisto SA, Clifford PR, Longabaugh R, et al. The relationship between abstinence for one year following pretreatment assessment and alcohol use and other functioning at two years in individuals presenting for alcohol treatment. J Stud Alcohol 2002;63:397–403.
14. Laudet A, Morgen K, White W. The role of social supports, spirituality, religiousness, life meaning and affiliation with 12-step fellowships in quality of life satisfaction among individuals in recovery from alcohol and drug use. Alcohol Treat Q 2006;24:33–74.
15. Pringle JL, Emptage NP, Hubbard RL. Unmet needs for comprehensive services in outpatient addiction treatment. J Subst Abuse Treat 2006;30:183–9.
16. Saitz R, Larson MJ, LaBelle C, et al. The case for chronic disease management for addiction. J Addict Med 2008;2:55–65.
17. McLellan AT, McKay JR, Forman R, et al. Reconsidering the evaluation of addiction treatment: from retrospective follow-up to concurrent recovery monitoring. Addiction 2005;100:447–58.
18. Miller WR, Rollnick S. Motivational interviewing: helping people change. 3rd edition. New York: Guilford Publications, Inc; 2012.
19. Mee-Lee D, Harrison J, Stawieray K. Tips and topics. Carson City (NV): The Change Companies; 2011.
20. McLellan AT, Luborsky L, Woody GE, et al. An improved diagnostic evaluation instrument for substance abuse patients. The addiction severity index. J Nerv Ment Dis 1980;168:26–33.
21. McLennan AT, Hagan TA, Levine M, et al. Supplemental social services improve ojutcomes in public addiction treatment. Addiction 1998;93:1489–99.
22. Hesse M, Vanderplassachen W, Rapp RC, et al. Case management for persons with substance use disorders. Cochrane Database Syst Rev 2007;(4):CD006265.

Use of Photovoice in Addiction

Gretchen Hope Miller Heery, FNP, BC, DrNP(c)

KEYWORDS

- Addiction • Images • Photographs • Photovoice • Recovery substance abuse

KEY POINTS

- Drug addiction is a major public health problem.
- Recovery is a challenging process of change for the addict that involves stigma.
- Photovoice provides an ability to address issues with a powerful visual image through clues to decode multiple layers of meaning within the addict's private world.

NATURE OF THE PROBLEM

Addiction to narcotic substances is an increasing public health problem.[1-3] The misuse of a drug is considered taking a medication different from that which was prescribed or for a different condition than prescribed.[1] It can cause harm to the individual, families, and community (**Table 1**).[1,4-8]

It is estimated that 4.4 million Americans chronically abuse drugs: 3.6 million are chronic cocaine users and 810,000 chronically use heroin (**Fig. 1**).[1,5,6,8–10] The National Survey on Drug Use and Health data noted illicit drug use in Americans older than age 12 to be second only to marijuana use. The number of persons with opioid dependence increased from 936,000 in 2002 to 1.4 million in 2011. An estimated 56.1% of opioid-dependent persons in 2011 were age 26 or older with a third (472,000) age 18 to 25. Illicit drug use has increased in teenagers and those older than age 50 by 50% between 2002 and 2011. There have been 1.9 million or more new nonmedical opioid users each year since 2002, contributing to increases in indicators of problems associated with its use.[7,8,11] In addition to illicit and controlled substance use, a national study identified an emerging trend in the abuse of prescription and over-the-counter drugs.[8,11]

There are enormous and increasing health care costs correlating to drug abuse caused by the lost productivity and increased medical requirements needed to treat severe drug-related health problems.[11] In 2011, the National Institutes of Health estimated that the financial costs of untreated opiate addiction are rising above $235 billion a year related to social costs of destroyed families, destabilized communities, increased health care costs, and increased crime.[4,5,8]

---

154 Semmels Hill Road, Lehighton, PA 18235, USA
E-mail address: heerychr@ptd.net

Nurs Clin N Am 48 (2013) 445–458
http://dx.doi.org/10.1016/j.cnur.2013.05.005
0029-6465/13/$ – see front matter © 2013 Elsevier Inc. All rights reserved.

Table 1
Harms of addiction

Individual	Community
Health	Reduced worker productivity
Disease	Increased rates of domestic violence
Poor parenting	Criminal behavior
Decreased self-esteem	Premature death
Increased public disorder	Morbidity
Poverty	Health care costs secondary to adverse
Increased police involvement and congestion in the courts	reactions and disease can also be seen

Data from Refs.[1,4–8]

ADDICTION

Recognizing the immediacy of reward associated with drug use coupled with the documented changes in brain chemistry that occur with long-term abuse of drugs is critically important to understanding why recovery can be difficult. Drug abuse is a disorder of the whole person. The problem is the person, not the drug. The addiction is only a symptom and not the essence of the disorder.[12] Addiction is a primary, chronic, neurobiologic disease, with genetic, psychosocial, and environmental factors influencing its development and manifestations (**Box 1**).[6,13–16] It is characterized by behaviors that include one or more of the following: impaired control over drug use, compulsive use, continued use despite harm, and craving.[13,17] It is medically diagnosed in the *Diagnostic and Statistical Manual of Mental Disorders, Fourth Edition — Text Revision* (**Table 2**).[1,17,18]

Research supports that those who misuse substances suffer from diffuse cortical damage,[14,16,19] most of which occurred in the frontal and temporal lobes. Although these addicts may seem to be able to function in everyday situations, loss of frontal brain activity limits one's executive ability leading to misinterpretations of actions. As a result, addictive people seem generally apathetic, indifferent, and lacking

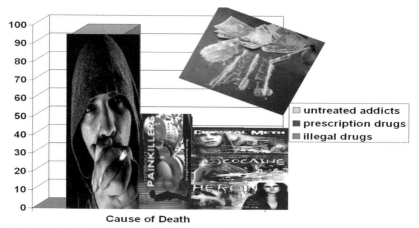

Fig. 1. Rates of addiction. (*Data from* Refs.[1,6,9,10]. Photos *courtesy of* Foundation for a Drug-Free World [www.drugfreeworld.org]; with permission.)

Box 1 Factors of addiction			
Neurobiologic	**Genetic**	**Psychosocial**	**Environmental**
Cortical damage of frontal and temporal lobes	Inherited	Problem avoidance (psychosis, stress, relationship issues)	Environment with drug available, unsafe Peer pressure

Data from Refs.[6,13–16]

initiative and spontaneity; show failure to organize or schedule work; and show a lack of sensitivity in social situations, such as emotional liability, outbursts of anger, caustic remarks, and insensitive behavior.[14,16] The stigma associated with the illness contributes to difficulty identifying, accessing, and continuing to stay and work on this illness in the needed treatment programs.[19]

RELAPSE

Drug and alcohol addicts can be expected to relapse 54% of the time according to studies.[8,11] Of this percentage, 61% relapse multiple times. It is common for addicts to relapse within 1 month after treatment. It is not unusual for addicts to relapse 12 months after treatment, and 47% relapse within the first year after treatment.[6,8] Relapse rates from addiction (40%–60%) can be compared with those suffering from other chronic illnesses, such as type I diabetes (30%–50%); hypertension (50%–70%); and asthma (50%–70%) (**Fig. 2**).[6] The same stigma is not attached to relapse of more socially acceptable diseases.

Addiction relapse is preventable. In 2011, 7.2 million persons older than age 12 were reported as needing treatment of addiction.[8,10] Of those that need treatment, 1.4 million persons have received treatment from a specialty facility. The remaining 5.8 million persons did not receive treatment despite 8.4% perceiving the need for treatment. Of these 488,000 persons without treatment, 61.6% reported that they made no

Table 2 DSM-IVR criteria	
Substance-Related Dependence	**Substance-Related Abuse**
Pattern of substance use leading to significant impairment in functioning	Consists of substance use history
One of the following must be present within a 12 mo period: 1. Recurrent use resulting in a failure to fulfill major obligations at work, school, or home; 2. Recurrent use in situations which are physically hazardous (eg, driving while intoxicated); 3. Legal problems resulting from recurrent use; or 4. Continued use despite significant social or interpersonal problems caused by the substance use.	1. Specific substance abuse; 2. Continuation of use despite related problems; 3. Increase in tolerance; and 4. Withdrawal symptoms.

Adapted from American Psychiatric Association. Diagnostic and Statistical Manual of Mental Disorders, Fourth Edition — Text Revision (DSMIV-TR) (2000). American Psychiatric Association: Arlington, VA.

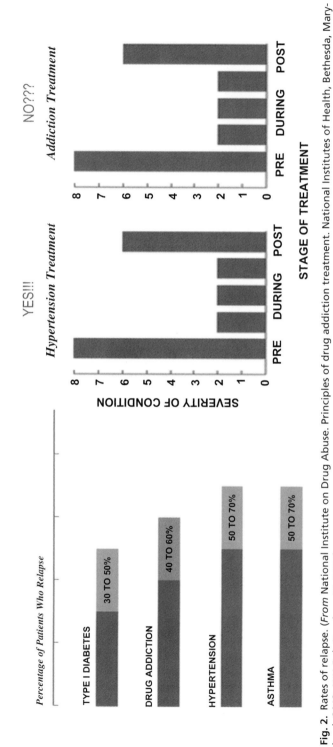
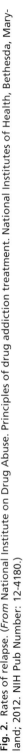

Fig. 2. Rates of relapse. (*From* National Institute on Drug Abuse. Principles of drug addiction treatment. National Institutes of Health, Bethesda, Maryland; 2012. NIH Pub Number: 12-4180.)

effort to seek treatment. The immediacy of reward associated with drug use clearly has some importance in understanding why recovery can be difficult. Understanding the process opioid-addicted adults use in recovery may possibly increase the rate of success in their recovery and lessen the effects drugs have on the population. Drug addiction should be treated like other chronic illnesses, with relapse indicating the need for renewed intervention. Addiction need not be a life sentence. Like other chronic diseases, it can be managed successfully.

RECOVERY

Recovery has been viewed as a continuous process containing benefits from lessons learned in treatment to consisting of multiple discontinuous stages to deliberate mindset changes. Some models are created based on the idea of recovery consisting of 6 to 10 stages (**Fig. 3**).[20,21] Boyarsky and McCance-Katz[4] describe recovery as a phase (**Fig. 4**). According to them it can "...best be conceptualized as a dynamic, fluid state that can shift from pre-conceptualization of substance modification on one end of the spectrum through the acute withdrawal or abstinence syndromes, early abstinence and extinction of symptoms (cravings) at the opposite end of the spectrum." According to other researchers, recovery is an opportunity for addicts to begin abstinence, change dysfunctional thinking and behavior, regain health, and in general reduce the chaos of substance abuse in their lives.[22–25]

Drug-addicted adults who are motivated to change are more successful in their recovery process.[6] Motivation is a complex and dynamic construct. It includes intrinsic and extrinsic dimensions (**Table 3**).[26,27] Research supports that there needs to be a transformation of extrinsic to intrinsic motivation of change to have long-term results. These tasks include developing a history of problems related to the addiction, recognizing a pattern of addiction-related problems, attempting to control its use, attempting abstinence without help, experiencing motivational crisis, and ending with agreeing to enter appropriate treatment.[24,26]

The Betty Ford Institute Consensus Panel does not support recovery as a specific method but as a personal condition (**Box 2**). Mindfulness, observing fears, anxiety, and compassion, must happen before recovery initiation.[26,28] Assessing attributes of recovery is a complex task, particularly in regard to the timing the improvement is measured, when recovery is determined, and when individuals are asked to identify the contributions of various factors of their recovery.

To date, recovery from addiction has been viewed from the perspective of policy makers and those without addiction. To understand the view and needs of those

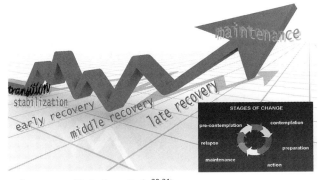

Fig. 3. Stages of recovery. (*Data from* Refs.[20,21])

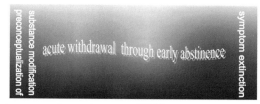

Fig. 4. Spectrum of recovery. (*Data from* Refs.[4,22–25])

afflicted with the disease and find the most effective treatment strategies it must be seen through the eyes of the addict. According to the National Institutes for Drug Abuse, research indicates that active participation in treatment is an essential component for optimal outcomes and can benefit even the most severely addicted individuals.[6] The primary goal of recovery is to change negative patterns of behavior, thinking, and feeling that predispose one to drug abuse.

PHOTOVOICE

Photovoice provides a community-based diagnostic tool to redress the inadequate theory on which programs may be based.[29] This method has the potential to offer a deeper perspective, insight, dimension of feeling, and perception in connecting with those who feel disconnected (**Box 3**).[29,30] It includes a process that uses cameras, film, discussion, and interaction. The written word provides a single view based on the writer's view. Photographs can emit feeling, emotion, and sometimes sensation with a simple glance, not just a single view. Photograph narration and versions have been used in all ages including preschoolers. A drug abuse addict may have difficulty expressing oneself well with the written word. It has been suggested that "the human brain processes stories more fully than other stimuli and they also note that impact is greater when the storyteller is recounting their own experience."[31] Photographs provide an accessible method to express the participant's thoughts about recovery.

PHOTOVOICE METHOD

Individuals use camera phones or digital cameras to record their recovery and document the photograph's meaning through documentation and discussion in a focus

Table 3	
Factors for recovery	
Intrinsic	**Extrinsic**
Will	Motivation to change, positive influences of family
Motivation: complex and dynamic construct	Legal pressures
Strength of religion and spirituality	Sanctions
More fundamental to the recovery process	Family pressures
Developing meaningful relationships	Initial positive urine drug screen
Replacing the addiction	External environment including dependency, health services, community, and sociopolitical issues
	Conventional lifestyles
	Better psychological support
	Relocation to drug free zone

Data from Refs.[24,26,27]

Box 2
Betty Ford's tasks for recovery

1. Series of tasks involving developing a history of problems related to addiction

2. Recognizing a pattern of addiction-related problems

3. Attempting to control its use

4. Attempting abstinence without help

5. Experiencing motivational crisis

6. Ending with agreeing to enter appropriate treatment

7. Mindfulness, observing fears, anxiety, and compassion, must happen before recovery initiation

Data from Refs.[26,28]

---

group format. Participants are asked to take photographs and discuss their experience with recovery from opioids. They are asked to include, from their everyday lives, photographs that are meaningful to them in explaining the how and why they are able to choose recovery to learn from the individual's impressions of what is recovery.

During the initial meeting, before starting the process, the lead person provides a verbal and written description of the process.[37–44] This process is to enhance internal reflection, self-awareness, and exchange of individual perceptions to initiate personal change. Reviewing photographic ethics and need for photograph release forms is important. Photographic instructions including outlining the parameters for creating

---

Box 3
Ten Benefits of Photovoice

1. Provides a voice to marginalized populations[32,33] and intends to reach policy makers and change policy design.

2. Provides an opportunity to describe the abstract, embedded within multi-layered meanings, without a reliance on words as the primary form of communication.

3. Provides an "insider's view to lay the groundwork for experimental knowledge construction."[34(p7)]

4. Provides an ability to address issues with a powerful visual image.

5. Provides a challenge for participants to examine their experience through deeper communication than verbal feedback because due to the image itself intercepts memory of the participant's experience.[35]

6. Does not require participants to be able to read or write and is not dependent on age, physical ability, or command of language.

7. Provides a sense of ownership and empowerment that can stimulate social action.[36–38]

8. Assists in the development of personal and social identities of the participants.

9. Provides a new opportunity of an environment of change through the combination of visual and narrative methods.

10. Provides clues to decode multiple layers of meaning within the participant's private world.[35]

Data from Refs.[29,32–38]

visual text and avoiding risky environments, identifiable images of people, instructions, or locations need to be reviewed. Information from observations, interviews, and pictures need to be held in the strictest of confidence.

The group discussion starts with a framing question, such as, "Tell me the story of what you've gone through, from being an active drug user to being where you are in the recovery process." Individuals can use cameras or camera phones and film to document salient issues and events in their recovery.[39–42] These photographs are printed. This assignment includes collecting images, sounds, and objects on film that represent ideas, emotions, and the journey toward recovery and change. Primarily presentation is through film and text, but the goal is to elicit the expressiveness of the individual. The individual may have a sound that keeps him or her in recovery, so this form can be included as to not limit experience to a two dimensional experience.

The next step of the process includes spending 1 week taking pictures with a camera and printing the photographs. Photographs are reflected on by the participants using SHOWED questions to guide thinking (**Fig. 5**). These questions are commonly used during picture telling or storytelling in Photovoice.[32,36,37,41,42,45] The individual narrows the photographs down to the six photographs that best describe their recovery. This process is to aid the individual in describing the six photographs that are the most significant and meaningful to the participant. This method helps to understand different perspectives and identify diversity and differences correlating to the influences that incite drug-addicted adults to choose recovery. This process involves correlating the individual personal characteristics, treatment attributes and choices, and environmental influences that affect the opioid addict's motivation to change and treatment, their entry into and subsequent engagement in a recovery method, and ultimately their recovery. The lead person can interject with probing questions to help generate discussion without leading the pattern.

Results from the first stage of photograph gathering and reflexive thought are processed into a second discussion group with others who are going through a similar situation using the same method.[32,36,37,41,42,45] In 2 to 3 weeks, or after all the pictures

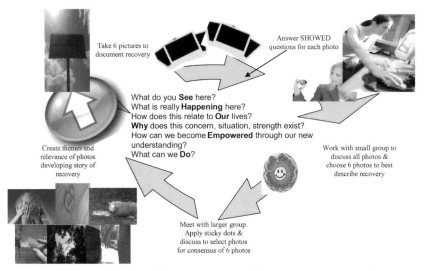

Take 6 pictures to document recovery

Answer SHOWED questions for each photo

What do you **See** here?
What is really **Happening** here?
How does this relate to **Our** lives?
Why does this concern, situation, strength exist?
How can we become **Empowered** through our new understanding?
What can we **Do**?

Create themes and relevance of photos developing story of recovery

Work with small group to discuss all photos & choose 6 photos to best describe recovery

Meet with larger group. Apply sticky dots & discuss to select photos for consensus of 6 photos

Fig. 5. Schematic of Photovoice. (Photos *courtesy of* iStockphoto.com, SmileMakers, Inc., and Foundation for a Drug-Free World [www.drugfreeworld.org]; with permission.)

from the participants are obtained, a second blogging week begins with the participants divided into three groups of like themes. During this week, the participant's interviews are digitally recorded through text; the photographers review written narratives from their cultural experiences that incorporate the images and learn collectively from the Photovoice experience. This session includes a five-step process. The steps include appreciating each other's photographs; small focus and blogging group work telling of the collective story; sharing of the story and photograph montage; and the sticky dot process (described later) formatted for computer use to organize the photographs based on the participant's evaluation. During this discussion period, participants select and tell stories about their pictures including the significance for their personal recovery from addiction. Participants are reminded to respect other's comments of the pictures. This is a process of information finding, to encourage reflection. The lead person constantly monitors the responses between participants and injects probing questions to keep the process on task for the best outcome. From the 30 photographs collected in the three groups, after further individual photograph discussion, six photographs are selected as a group consensus that best describes their voice. The group creates a team photograph board that expresses one common voice allowing reflection and feedback.

In the next couple weeks, other participants in the study have the opportunity to also comment and reflect on the photographs and their perception of the meaning toward recovery. The other participants in the Photovoice process participate through facilitated discussion boards and analysis.[32,36,37,41,42,45] The process continues through multiple boards and reorganization of the photographs to allow others to appreciate the photos and join in multiple discussion boards to further discuss and develop the picture through concrete to cultural to abstract meaning. During the week, each participant is given 10 colored dots to attach to pictures as directed (sticky dot process). Each color dot represents a theme created from the previous discussion. The participants review the new themes and "place" the corresponding dots on the picture they believe speaks the best to the overall theme and purpose of the group. The dot markers are not be revealed to the other participants until everyone has made their selections. During the next week, the lead person counts the dots and groups the most popular photographs in each category into a first round gallery layout. These are displayed for continued discussion throughout the following week.

Finally, the photographs are organized through a group consensus of six pictures. The information obtained from the discussion boards, written comments, and photographs are coded and evaluated using probing questions including the SHOWED acronym consistent with the Photovoice method (see **Fig. 5**). The participants share their individual and collective experiences as related to specific photographs, naming underlying themes and revising and reinventing groupings, creating community relevance. The participants choose the pictures they want to present, tell the story of the picture through contextualization, and discuss its meaning and importance.[34,36,37,39,43,44,46] Then the participants code the themes to formulate theories and potentially present to policy makers during the focus group.

The close of these discussions includes questions of what was learned about self, group, and community; what the next steps are; and who needs to hear their voice. Because of the sensitive and stigmatized nature of the concept of addiction and recovery, hotline numbers and a referral name and number are provided to all participants. These are provided to allow for crisis access if relapse or anxiety develops during this process. It is beneficial for the recovering addict to be engaged in the process while learning and teaching about pattern recognition and problem avoidance in their own recovery journey.[33,37,44,45]

Table 4
Limitations

Limitations	Precautions
Privacy	Acknowledge and release forms Private discussion areas
Confidentiality/stigma	Acknowledge and release forms Videos presenting issues related to confidentiality Crisis hotline provided Voluntary participation Only participants have access to discussion, photographs
Consent	Authority and responsibility discussions Ethical consent signed Photography consent signed Thoughts toward context and content of photographs
Misrepresentation	Videos presenting issues related to appropriateness of photographs Avoid disclosure of embarrassing and personal facts of individual Advised not to take photographs of faces or placing a person at risk or in false light No photographs of private people or private places
Safety	Video of safety issues Have ability to leave study at any time "Street sense" Present in alternative ways, such as abstract representation
Ownership of photographs	Photographs are owned by the photographer
Bias	Through the eyes of the beholder What is photographed, chosen, and written is at the discretion of the participant
Limit of full context of information	Data coded by participants
Limited to recovering addicts	Participants are active in recovery program, which is overseen by a provider
Cost of supplies	Limited to photography
Participant reviewed	Probing questions injected as needed Monitored discussion Consistent with the process for Photovoice Description of photo; Why do you want to share this photo; What is the real story the photo tells and how does it relate to your life and the lives of people in your community or both
Vulnerable population	Photovoice used on all ages Population comfortable with using social media Participants choose pictures they want to present The effectiveness of work is based on bonds of trust and commitment that participant stories and voices are meaningful

Data from Refs.[29,36,39,42,43,45,46]

LIMITATIONS OF PHOTOVOICE

Limitations of photographic data include objectifying a specific time and place under specific circumstances that might or might not be ideal for capturing the essence of what it is trying to represent (**Table 4**).[46] The angle of the picture remains static providing one direction. Some ethical issues related to this method include privacy, confidentiality, consent, misrepresentation, safety, ownership of the actual photographs, and potential for voyeurism.[36,39,42,43] An element of bias is a potential because of the choice of pictures or ability of the facilitator to influence pictures. The cost of supplies because of the requirements of cameras, access to private secure computer and Internet, and delivery methods available (direct download vs SD card and mail) may affect ability to participate. In addition, the time between when a photograph is taken, interviews, and limitation of the full context of the action may cause some constraints.[29,42,43,45]

USE OF PHOTOVOICE WITH ADDICTION

Understanding the process of recovery from drug abuse creates an opportunity to maintain socially acceptable behaviors, and decrease the risk of participating in illegal activities and making poor choices. Participants may have a more difficult time expressing their thoughts in written words but may be more expressive through creative thought. The use of Photovoice provides an open, creative environment to unearth recovery attributes. Photovoice can help the individual with pattern recognition and problem avoidance by asking the individual to record what he or she perceives as important in his or her personal recovery process. This method can aid the participant to elicit the unknown within the known and understand the "hidden consciousness of their experiences."[35(p10)] It can provide an opportunity to describe the abstract, embedded within multilayered meanings, without a reliance on words as the primary form of communication. Through the use of cameras, the addict can record their recovery, document the photographs' meaning, and learn what influences him or her to choose recovery.

Davidson and colleagues[35] describe visual images as having "...the capacity of bypassing cognitive defenses of our experiences to tap directly into our emotional and spiritual/intuitive zones of consciousness." It provides an "...insider's view to lay the groundwork for experimental knowledge construction."[34(pp7),37,45] Photovoice also provides an ability to address issues with a powerful visual image.[46,47] These visual images can challenge participants to examine their experience through deeper communication than verbal feedback. The image has the ability to intercept the memory of the participant's experience over the verbal word.[35,46,47] It does not require participants to be able to read or write and is not dependent on age, physical ability, or command of language. This combination of visual and narrative methods provides a new opportunity for an environment of change.

SUMMARY

This method may be beneficial for the recovering addict to be engaged in a process while learning and teaching others, such as a health care team or stakeholders, about pattern recognition and problem avoidance in their own recovery journey. It is a process of providing six pictures that support the individual's process of recovery, commenting on the photographs through reflective thought using SHOWED questions, looking at other's photographs in the group, and continually reducing the number of photographs by regrouping themes to the six best photographs that fit the group's idea of recovery. To understand the view and needs of those afflicted with addiction, recovery must be seen through the eyes of those recovering.

REFERENCES

1. Denisco RA, Chandler RK, Compton WM. Addressing the intersecting problems of opioid misuse and chronic pain treatment. Exp Clin Psychopharmacol 2008; 16(5):417–28.
2. Katz N. Opioids: after thousands of years, still getting to know you. Clin J Pain 2007;23(4):303–6.
3. Musto D. The mystery of addiction. Lancet 1999;354(Suppl):SIV1.
4. Boyarsky BK, McCance-Katz EF. Improving the quality of substance dependency treatment with pharmacotherapy. Subst Use Misuse 2000;35(12–14):2095–125.
5. Nationwide trends. More information. 2012. Available at: www.drugabuse.gov/publications/drugfacts/nationwide-trends. Accessed March 4, 2013.
6. National Institute Drug Abuse. National Institute of Health, Bethesda, MD. More information available at: http://www.nida.nih.gov/PODAT/faqs.html. Accessed July 19, 2010.
7. Price AM, Ilgen MA, Bohnert AS. Prevalence and correlates of nonmedical use of prescription opioids in patients seen in a residential drug and alcohol treatment program. J Subst Abuse Treat 2011;41:208–14.
8. Substance Abuse and Mental Health Services Administration. Results from the 2011 National Survey on Drug Use and Health: summary of national findings. NSDUH series H-44, HHS Publication No. SMH 12–4713. Rockville (MD): SAMHSA; 2012. Available at: http://www.samhsa.gov/data/NSDUH/2k11Results/NSDUHresults2011.htm. Accessed March 15, 2012.
9. Healthy People 2010 substance abuse. Available at: http://www.healthypeople.gov/document/html/volume2/26substance.htm#_Toc489757831. Accessed March 15, 2012.
10. Mendelson J, Flower K, Pletcher MJ, et al. Addiction to prescription opioids: characteristics of the emerging epidemic and treatment with buprenorphine. Exp Clin Psychopharmacol 2008;16(5):435–41.
11. Centers for Disease Control Prevention. 2012. Available at: http://www.cdc.gov/mmwr/preview/mmwrhtml/mm5745a3.htm. Assessed March 5, 2013.
12. DeLeon G. Integrative recovery: a stage paradigm. Subst Abuse 1996;17(1): 51–63.
13. American Society of Addiction Medicine. Definition of addiction. 2011. Available at: http://www.asam.org/for-the-public/definition-of-addiction. Accessed August 26, 2011.
14. Cristo G. The role of neuropsychology in substance misuse treatment. J Subst Misuse 1998;3:61–6.
15. Feltenstein MW, See RE. The neurocircuitry of addiction: an overview. Br J Pharmacol 2008;154(2):261–74.
16. Robles E, Huang BE, Simpson PM, et al. Delay discounting, impulsiveness, and addiction severity in opioid-dependent patients. J Subst Abuse Treat 2011;41: 354–62.
17. American Psychiatric Association. Diagnostic and statistical manual of mental disorders. Washington (DC): American Psychiatric Association; 1994.
18. Diagnostic and statistical manual of mental disorders, fourth edition — text revision. Arlington (VA): American Psychiatric Association; 2000.

19. Barretto RP, Ko TH, Jung JC, et al. Time-lapse imaging of disease progression in deep brain areas using fluorescence microendoscopy. Nat Med 2011;17:223–8.
20. Prochaska JO, DiClemente CC, Norcross JC. In search of how people change: applications to addictive behaviors. Am Psychol 1992;47:1102–14.
21. Darbo N. Alternative diversion programs for nurses with impaired practice: completers and non-completers. J Addict Nurs 2005;16:169–85.
22. Schwarzer R, Luszcynska A. How to overcome health-compromising behaviors: the health action process approach. Eur Psychol 2008;13:141–51.
23. Clarke S, Oades LG, Crowe TP. Recovery in mental health: a movement toward wellbeing & meaning in contrast to an avoidance of symptoms. Psychiatr Rehabil J 2012;35(4):297–304.
24. Richert J, Schuz N, Schuz B. Stages of health behavior change and mindsets: a latent class approach. Health Psychol 2013;32(3):273–82.
25. Schuz B, Sniehottaa FF, Mallach N, et al. Predicting transitions from preintentional, intentional and actional stages of change. Health Educ Res 2009;24:64–75.
26. Nordfjaern T, Rundmo T, Hole R. Treatment and recovery as perceived by patients with substance addiction. J Psychiatr Ment Health Nurs 2010;17:46–64.
27. Vakili S, Currie S, el-Guebaly N. Evaluating the utility of drug testing in an outpatient addiction program. Addic Disord Their Treat 2009;8(1):22–32.
28. Betty Ford Institute Consensus Panel. What is recovery? A working definition from the Betty Ford Institute. J Subst Abuse Treat 2007;33:221–8.
29. Wang C, Burris MA. Photovoice: concept, methodology and use of participatory needs assessment. Health Educ Behav 1997;24(3):369–87.
30. Marinak BA, Strickland MJ, Keat JB. Using photo-narration to support all learners. Young Child 2010;65(5):32–8.
31. Lillyman S, Gutteridge R, Berridge P. Using storyboarding technique in the classroom to address end of life experiences in practice and engage student nurses in deeper reflection. Nurse Educ Pract 2011;11:179–85.
32. Fleming J, Mahoney J, Carlson E, et al. An ethnographic approach to interpreting a mental illness Photovoice exhibit. Arch Psychiatr Nurs 2009;23(1):16–24.
33. Sharma M. Photovoice in alcohol and drug education. J Alcohol Drug Educ 2010; 54(1):3–6.
34. Chircop A, Sheppard-LeMoine D. Photonovella and Photovoice: two innovative research methods of data collection and beyond. Theoria 2004;13(3):4–9.
35. Davidson J, Dottin JW Jr, Penna SL, et al. Visual sources and the qualitative research dissertation: ethics, evidence and the politics of academia. Moving innovation in higher education from the center to the margins. IJEA 2009;10(27). Available at: http://www.ijea.org/v10n27/. Accessed February 21, 2012.
36. Goodhart FW, Hsu J, Baek JH, et al. A view through a different lens: Photovoice as a tool for student advocacy. J Am Coll Health 2006;55:53–6.
37. Hergenrather KC, Rhodes SD, Cowan CA, et al. Photovoice as a community-based participatory research: a qualitative review. Am J Health Behav 2009; 33(6):686–98.
38. Wang CC, Morrell-Samuels S, Hutchinson P, et al. Flint Photovoice: community-building among youth, adults, and policy makers. Am J Public Health 2004; 94(6):911–3.
39. Cook K, Buck G. Photovoice: a community-based socioscientific pedagogical tool. Sci Scope 2010;33(7):35–8.
40. Vengus J, Glen S, MacKenzie L. Photovoice: Hamilton Youth Project. Project in community. 2008. Available at: http://www.photovoice.ca. Accessed March 15, 2012.

41. Wang CC. Photovoice: a participatory action research strategy applied to women's health. J Womens Health 1999;8(2):185–92.
42. Wang CC, Redwood-Johnson YA. Photovoice ethics: perspectives from Flint Photovoice. Health Educ Behav 2001;28(5):560–72.
43. Castleden H, Garvin T, Nation HF. Modifying Photovoice for community based participatory indigenous research. Soc Sci Med 2008;66:1393–405.
44. Baker TA, Wang CC. Photovoice: use of a participatory action research method to explore the chronic pain experience in older adults. Qual Health Res 2006;16(10): 1405–13.
45. Carlson ED, Engebretson J, Chamberlain RM. Photovoice as a social process of critical consciousness. Qual Health Res 2006;16(6):836–52.
46. Hagarty DE, Clark DJ. Using imagery and storytelling to educate outpatients about 12-step programs and improve their participation in community-based programs. J Addict Nurs 2009;20:86–92.
47. Ruby LW. Layers of seeing and seeing through layers: the work of art in the age of digital imagery. J Aesthetic Educ 2008;42(2):51–6.

Peer Assistance for Nurses with Substance-Use Disorders

Albert Rundio Jr, PhD, DNP, RN, APRN, CARN-AP, NEA-BC[a,b,c,*]

KEYWORDS

- Substance use • Nurse • Peer assistance • Addiction

KEY POINTS

- Addictions can be prevalent among health professionals, owing to access and their understanding of pharmacologic function.
- State laws on medication abuse and theft by health professionals vary greatly.
- Peer-assistance programs may help nurses who abuse substances to receive treatment and maintain licensure.

When we think of substance-use disorders, we tend to think of the general population and not those in the health professions. It is important to recognize that substance-use disorder crosses all boundaries: economic, educational, gender, geographic, employment status, and others. The reality is that addictions can be very prevalent in the health professions, as these individuals are intelligent and know how drugs function. One of the other key factors is that those in the health professions generally have easy access to medications and controlled substances. To date many systems have been implemented in attempts to prevent nurses and other providers from abusing drugs; for example, computerized automated delivery systems of medication. Nevertheless, substance-use disorders are still prevalent in the health professions, and one cannot exclude these professionals from any discussion on substance use.

It is important to understand that each state within the United States is an independent entity. Thus nursing practice, rules, and regulations vary from state to state. For example, some states are very punitive when a nurse has a substance-use disorder, and may even remove the person's license for a set period of time until the nurse is engaged fully in recovery and demonstrates no relapse or remission. Other states attempt to support the nurse without the nurse losing licensure while the nurse is under

[a] College of Nursing & Health Professions, Drexel University, 1505 Race Street, Room #429, Philadelphia, PA 19102, USA; [b] International Nurses Society on Addictions, PO Box 14846, Lenexa, KS 66285-4846, USA; [c] Lighthouse at Mays Landing, 5034 Atlantic Avenue, Mays Landing, NJ 08330, USA
* Corresponding author. College of Nursing & Health Professions, Drexel University, 1505 Race Street, Room #429, Philadelphia, PA 19102.
E-mail address: aar27@drexel.edu

Nurs Clin N Am 48 (2013) 459–463
http://dx.doi.org/10.1016/j.cnur.2013.05.002
0029-6465/13/$ – see front matter © 2013 Elsevier Inc. All rights reserved.

treatment and beyond. As substance-use disorder is a disease process, those states that have excellent peer-assistance programs tend to be the most successful in getting nurses immersed in recovery as well as maintaining their licensure and employment as a nurse. Some nurses who enter such programs are not successful as they are not compliant with the peer-assistance program's recommendations, and therefore risk loss of licensure for set time periods.

Each state has its own method of implementing the peer-assistance program. For example, a state board of nursing may contract with an agency that conducts peer assistance. An agency is generally selected by a process known as competitive bidding. Contracts are awarded for a defined time period, for example, 5 years. Many agencies will also seek grant funding related to peer assistance and substance-use disorders. There is also a national association that meets annually to discuss peer assistance. In general, the agency appoints a not-for-profit board of directors to oversee the functioning of the agency, and will also employ legal counsel. The agency will make periodic reports to the respective state board of nursing. Funds are allocated by state legislation to run the peer-assistance program, along with grant funding. A comprehensive program will include intense monitoring of the nurse for relapse; for example, monthly analysis of urine specimens to monitor drug use. The program will also include individual and group counseling sessions and usually mandatory attendance at 12-step meetings. In collaboration with the respective state board of nursing, the agency will define time parameters for how long the nurse must remain in the program; for example, a state may mandate that a nurse be in the program for 3 years. Some states require a longer period (eg, 5 years) for certified registered nurse anesthetists to remain in the program. A good peer-assistance program will maintain excellent data on the number of nurses entered into the program, and the number of nurses that complete the program successfully and maintain recovery.

Legislation entitled the American with Disabilities Act of 1990[1] drastically changed the approach of state boards of nursing to dealing with nurses who have substance-use disorders. When nurses are engaged in treatment they are protected by this Act,[1] and the state board of nursing cannot remove their license. In truth the Act[1] has triggered state boards of nursing to engage in more peer-assistance activities rather than punitive ones, which is very positive for the profession, as nurses who engage in recovery continue to hold their license and are able to return to employment.

As an aid to explanation, 3 case studies are reported.

CASE STUDY 1

Nurse anesthetists and anesthesiologists are one of the groups of professionals who have easy access to controlled substances. Providers each have their own anesthesia cart, basically having control of the substances in the cart. It is therefore easy for these providers to divert medication, namely, controlled substances.

JD is employed as a certified registered nurse anesthetist. JD has always had a somewhat nasty attitude. JD is married to a nurse and has a couple of children. The operating room (OR) staff has noticed that for the past few months JD has been losing weight. The OR staff makes the assumption that JD must have AIDS, as he is a male nurse and must be gay or bisexual.

The nursing director at this acute-care hospital is notified by the director of pharmacy. The director of pharmacy reports to the nursing director that the use of Sublimaze has doubled in the OR. The nursing director questions the pharmacy director as to whether there has been a change in anesthesia practice; for example, is double the amount of Sublimaze now being used on patients? The pharmacy director reports that there has not been a practice change in anesthesia. The nursing director then asks if the number of OR cases has increased. The pharmacy director states that there has been no increase. The nursing director then tells the pharmacy director that she suspects that someone is diverting and using Sublimaze in the OR. The pharmacy director confirms this assumption. The nursing director then questions the pharmacy director: "do you have an idea of who this is?" The pharmacy director replies that he has no idea as to the identity.

Based on this information, the nursing director notifies the state's drug enforcement agency (DEA) requesting an investigation. The DEA responds by sending an investigator to the acute-care facility. Within about 1 week of investigation, the investigator is able to identify the nurse anesthetist as the person who is diverting Sublimaze.

Memorial Day weekend follows the investigator's discovery. There is a 3-day holiday, and the investigator returns to the acute-care facility on Tuesday. He reviews the obstetric records to ascertain if any cesarean sections have been completed over the weekend. He checks the OR and the anesthesia log books, and discovers that 3 patients were signed out by the nurse anesthetist in question for receiving Sublimaze for 3 cesarean sections over the weekend when no such surgeries occurred. The investigator is now 100% sure that the nurse anesthetist is diverting, and most likely using, the Sublimaze.

The investigator contacts the nursing director with his discovery and advises her that he wants to schedule a confrontation with the nurse anesthetist for that Thursday. He advises the nursing director that another investigator will be with him when he confronts the nurse anesthetist. He states that it is the role of the nursing director to call the nurse anesthetist down to her office. She will introduce the nurse anesthetist to the investigators and will then leave, to allow the investigators the opportunity to question the nurse anesthetist.

On Thursday the nurse anesthetist is confronted by the DEA investigators. The nurse anesthetist admits that he had been diverting and using Sublimaze in the hospital while doing cases. He states that he would go to another nursing floor in the bathroom and use the Sublimaze between cases, as his habit had increased dramatically secondary to the development of more tolerance.

The investigator consults with the nurse director and advises her that it took 2 hours of questioning the nurse anesthetist about their suspicions before the nurse anesthetist finally admitted he had been diverting and abusing Sublimaze.

In this particular state, the nurse anesthetist lost his license for a 3-year time period. This nurse anesthetist was also licensed in another state, where he did not lose his license because he was entered into a peer-assistance monitoring program for a 5-year period, as was the rule in that state. This nurse anesthetist did very well in the peer-assistance monitoring program after an initial 28-day treatment program followed by an intensive outpatient treatment program. After immersion in the peer-assistance program, counseling and group meetings, and monitoring, the nurse anesthetist was able to return to work.

CASE STUDY 2

MJ is a nurse employed in a physical rehabilitation center. MJ has had a problem using benzodiazepines. Her use pattern has increased secondary to tolerance. Another nurse on her unit recognizes that patients who should be more sedate are not. She reports this to the director of nursing, who in turn reports this to the pharmacy director. A review of records demonstrates that when the patients are most awake, MJ is the nurse administering the benzodiazepines. The nursing director concludes that MJ is diverting the medication. The nursing director confronts MJ along with the nursing supervisor as a witness. MJ readily confesses that she has been diverting the benzodiazepines for her own use. The nursing director realizes that if MJ is reported to the state board of nursing before she enters treatment, she will have her nursing license terminated. The nursing director gives MJ an alternative: she must enter a 28-day treatment program, followed by an intensive outpatient program. The nursing director advises her that if she does this, she will maintain her job and will not be reported to the board of nursing. The nurse readily accepts this offer and enters the 28-day inpatient treatment program for substance-use disorders. The nurse does well in treatment and then agrees to an intensive outpatient program as well as monitoring by the facility.

In this case there are problems regarding the way in which the situation was handled by the director of nursing. Substance-use disorders constitute an offense reportable to the board of nursing, meaning that the person who discovers the nurse who was abusing drugs, but does not report the offense, could also be held culpable. The director has no real means knowing what the nurse is doing on the outside. Even though addictions have a great many outcomes, some individuals do continue to relapse, and use drugs despite the consequences. The better approach here would have been to certainly get the nurse who was diverting and using drugs into treatment, but also to report the nurse to the respective state board of nursing so that she could be monitored continuously by the board, which would help maintain her recovery. This strategy would also protect the nursing director's license, should MJ relapse.

CASE STUDY 3

BJ is an licensed practical nurse (LPN) employed in an acute-care hospital on the maternity unit. As an LPN in this US state, BJ is licensed to administer oral medication. The vast majority of postdelivery patients on this unit have Percocet ordered for a specified time period.

The nurse manager of the maternity unit identifies that reels of Percocet are missing when the narcotic count is completed. She reports this to the pharmacy director, who in turn notifies the director of nursing. The pharmacy director conducts a preliminary investigation but is unable to identify the culprit nurse. The nursing director decides to ask the DEA to investigate.

A new investigator from the DEA is sent to the facility. After a preliminary investigation, the nursing director meets with the investigator to discuss his findings. The nursing director advises the investigator that she suspects BJ is the culprit. The investigator advises the nursing director that he is in agreement. The nursing director questions the investigator as to when he plans to confront her. He advises the nursing director that he is not yet ready to confront the nurse, as he is only 95% certain that this person is the nurse diverting the Percocet and that he needs to be 100% certain before confrontation.

BJ is admitted to the acute-care facility with abdominal pain. A surgical consult is done, and the surgeon determines that her gallbladder needs to be removed. BJ's insurance requires prior approval for surgery. The physician at the insurance company reviews the case and BJ's medical record, and cannot find a medical reason for doing the gallbladder surgery. He denies approval of the gallbladder surgery. BJ then advises the surgeon and her attending physician that she has been abusing Percocet. The attending physician consults the addictions specialist at the hospital. He evaluates BJ and determines that she needs inpatient treatment at a detoxification center. BJ is then transferred for inpatient care at a local substance-abuse treatment center, which occurs over the weekend.

The director of nursing reports to work on Monday and learns what has happened to BJ. She then notifies the investigator and advises him that his 95% suspicion is now 100% and that BJ has been transferred and admitted to a treatment center over the weekend. As BJ is in treatment, under the American with Disabilities Act 1990[1] her nursing license cannot be terminated. The investigator advises the director of nursing that he will report his findings as well as these occurrences to the respective state board of nursing. BJ does well in the 28-day treatment program. She then attends an intensive outpatient program for 1 month, and is permitted by the board of nursing to return to work. The decision is made to return her to the maternity unit, as she worked day shift and the nursing manager was aware of what had occurred. BJ is not allowed to administer narcotics for a 1-year period. The nursing director receives quarterly reporting forms from the board of nursing, to which she has to report on BJ's progress. BJ progresses nicely for around 9 months, and all reports to the board of nursing are positive.

After about 9 months of monitoring BJ's performance, the nursing director is called by a pharmacist from a retail pharmacy in the general locale. The pharmacist advises the nursing director that he had to have one of her nurses arrested. BJ had been arrested for writing prescriptions for Percocet and floating them to various pharmacies within the geographic region. When investigated, it was discovered that BJ sought employment at one of the hospitals' gynecologist offices during evening hours. BJ had lifted one of the gynecologist prescription pads and was writing Percocet prescriptions for herself. Now that BJ was under arrest and not in treatment, the state board of nursing removed her license for a 3-year period.

This final case demonstrates why reporting to the respective state board of nursing and having proper monitoring is critical for the protection of patients and also for the protection of nursing as a profession.

REFERENCE

1. American with Disabilities Act of 1990. Available at: http://lac.org/doc_library/lac/publications/ada.pdf. Accessed May 12, 2013.

Monitoring Nurses with Substance-Use Disorders in New Jersey

Jamie Smith, MSN, RN, CCRN

KEYWORDS

- Nurse • Substance abuse • New Jersey • Addiction

KEY POINTS

- As many as 6% to 8% of nurses are estimated to abuse alcohol or other substances.
- Monitoring and peer-assistance programs have been created to increase the understanding of abuse, to support nurses in their recovery and safe return to practice, and to protect public safety.
- In New Jersey, the Recovery and Monitoring Program (RAMP) and Peer Assistance Program exist, whose goals are to protect patients and to support nurses during their recovery and successful return to nursing practice.

Substance abuse and addiction among nurses is a significant problem, with consequences that are far reaching and frequently devastating. The estimates of nurses who abuse alcohol and other substances vary depending on the source, but range from between 6% and 8% up to nearly 15%.[1] Despite the prevalence of this disease, stigma and misunderstanding exist within the nursing profession and health care system. Nurses have additional risk factors for developing substance-use disorders in their workplace, and face challenges unique to their role when returning to work.

Over the last few decades, monitoring programs and peer-assistance programs have developed to increase our understanding of this phenomenon. These programs are designed to support nurses during their recovery and safe return to practice, and, most importantly, to protect public safety.[2] In New Jersey, the Recovery and Monitoring Program (RAMP) and Peer Assistance Program exist, whose goals are to protect patients and to support nurses during their recovery and successful return to nursing practice.

YESTERDAY

The Peer Assistance Program was initiated in 1980 by a small group of dedicated addiction nurses. After witnessing colleagues in throes of substance-abuse disorders,

New Jersey State Nurses Association, 1479 Pennington Road, Trenton, NJ 08618, USA
E-mail address: jamie@njsna.org

Nurs Clin N Am 48 (2013) 465–468
http://dx.doi.org/10.1016/j.cnur.2013.05.003
0029-6465/13/$ – see front matter © 2013 Elsevier Inc. All rights reserved.

spiraling toward disaster without appropriate help, these nurses began holding peer-assistance meetings. One nurse at a time joined the voluntary meetings, offering each other support as they found their way. Given the occupational hazards of health care professions, the groups focused on recovery through a framework of nursing. Since those early days the program has had the motto "Nurses Supporting Nurses."

The Peer Assistance Program sought to help one nurse at a time through support groups, but more far-reaching changes were needed to make a difference within the larger nursing community. The New Jersey State Nurses Association sought support for this program from the New Jersey Board of Nursing and Department of Health and Senior Services. By 1988, the Peer Assistance Program had received grant funding to provide education, expand support groups and staff, and open a 24-hour hotline for nurses in need of help.

As the years passed, the Peer Assistance Program grew in size and scope. Providing New Jersey with expertise on impaired nursing practice, the Peer Facilitators, as they are now called, represent nursing throughout New Jersey on committees, in the workplace, and with speaking engagements. The program holds nearly 25 support groups and continues to grow to meet the needs of the nurses in New Jersey. The support groups provide support in recovery and professional issues, and assist in reentry to nursing practice.

Regulatory changes were needed to reduce the barriers in early identification of nurses in need of help. In the 1980s and 1990s, the approach of the New Jersey Board of Nursing was disciplinary in nature. Unfortunately, disciplinary-only approaches can prevent the timely removal of nurses from practice, thereby delaying treatment.[2] The fear of disciplinary and legal action prevented many nurses from seeking help. Because of regulatory processes, the disciplinary approach and legal process may be cumbersome and long. Sullivan and colleagues found that it took up to 3 years to remove an impaired nurse from practice with a disciplinary model.[3]

Alternatives to disciplinary approaches advocate for early intervention, removal from practice, monitoring, and reentry into the workplace. There are several alternative approaches to discipline, but overall they share the following features: a contract, expectation to complete appropriate treatment, participation in a support group, random drug screenings, workplace monitoring, and abstinence from controlled substances. In return for compliance in the program, the nurse has the opportunity to avoid public disciplinary action.[1]

The New Jersey State Nurses Association began advocating for changes to the Nurse Practice Act to allow for an alternative to discipline in 1997. The New Jersey State Nurses Association in cooperation with the New Jersey Board of Nursing began developing the infrastructure for the monitoring program known as RAMP. RAMP began accepting nurses in 2003 while still a pilot program. In 2005, the New Jersey State Legislature passed changes to the practice act and established the Alternative to Discipline Program for nurses (NJ 45:11-24.10).

TODAY

RAMP is a private, voluntary program that offers nurses support in receiving the appropriate treatment, closely monitoring their recovery. RAMP is an example of an Alternative to Discipline Program administered by the Institute for Nursing, the foundation of the New Jersey State Nurses Association, in collaboration with the New Jersey Board of Nursing. This type of program provides a balance between public protection and the nurse's rights. The goals of the program are to ensure both the safety of the public and the health of the nursing workforce. It provides nurses with treatment referrals and monitoring related to their recovery and reentry into practice, while the Board provides oversight. The participation of nurses is private as long as they remain compliant; in the case of noncompliance, nurses are referred to the Board for disciplinary action.[1]

Nurses are referred to RAMP by employers, colleagues, the Board, and the nurses themselves. Nurses enter into an individualized agreement with the program that includes all requirements. RAMP monitoring includes random urine drug screens, monthly self-reports, attendance at 12-step and peer-support meetings, return-to-work oversight, and employment monitoring. The nurses are expected to remain free of controlled substances and to submit any prescriptions to the program. Nurses must undergo 5 years of monitoring and at least 6 months of practice before being eligible to complete RAMP.

Returning to practice is often the first issue raised by a nurse when being referred to RAMP. The nurses participating in RAMP are required to refrain from practicing until they complete appropriate treatment, demonstrate a period of sobriety, and are properly prepared to practice. The program evaluates nurses through a collaborative return-to-work process. Nurses must present their plan for returning to work and maintain sobriety within their peer support group. The support groups, peer facilitator, RAMP case manager, and any other treatment provider offer input on the decision and additional work restrictions. Work restrictions are individualized, but always include the mandatory disclosure of nurses' participation in RAMP to their direct supervisor, monthly reports from the supervisor on practice, and continuation of RAMP monitoring. Approximately 40% of nurses enrolled in RAMP are currently working in nursing.

TOMORROW

The profession of nursing and, in particular, nursing in New Jersey has made momentous strides in providing our colleagues with respectful care and improving patient safety. The adoption of an Alternative to Discipline Program was a regulatory triumph for nurses. However, there is a continued need to reverse the "throwaway nurse syndrome" that still exists within health care organizations and, in some cases, within nursing.[4,5] The stigma that exists regarding nurses in recovery must be addressed. In today's changing health care environment, we need every good nurse we have. RAMP and the Peer Assistance Program are striving to educate nurses, administrations, and the public about substance abuse and are encouraging prevention, intervention, and monitoring.

For the nursing profession to meet the growing needs in health care, we must be prepared to care for each other in the best way possible. Nurses and all health care workers must have a just, fair environment that treats substance-use disorders as the medical diagnosis it is. Stigma will simply lead to secrecy and severe consequences to both patients and the profession. Supportive work environments, beginning with leadership, can and must create a culture of understanding, support, and transparency, which will promote patient safety.[1] No one should suffer the burden of substance abuse or mental illness alone. The Peer Assistance Forum and Recovery and Monitoring Program are available to offer help and support to nurses in New Jersey.

REFERENCES

1. National Council of State Boards of Nursing. Substance use disorder in nursing: a resource manual and guidelines for alternative and disciplinary monitoring programs. 2011. Available at: http://www.ncsbn.org. Accessed April 20, 2013.

2. Monroe T, Pearson F, Kenaga H. Procedures for handling cases of substance abuse among nurses: a comparison of disciplinary and alternative programs. J Addict Nurs 2008;19:159–61.
3. Sullivan E, Bissell L, Leffler D. Drug use and disciplinary actions among 300 nurses. Int J Addict 1990;25:375–91.
4. Darbro N. Alternative diversion programs for nurses with impaired practice: completers and noncompleters. J Addict Nurs 2005;16(4):169–85.
5. Darbro N. Overview of issues related to coercion and monitoring in alternative diversion programs for nurses: a comparison to drug courts: part 2. J Addict Nurs 2009;20(1):24–33.

Health Promotion and Prevention Strategies

Kathleen Bradbury-Golas, DNP, RN, NP-C, ACNS-BC[a,b,*]

KEYWORDS

- Health promotion • Recovery • Opiate addiction • Relapse prevention

KEY POINTS

- The overuse of alcohol and illicit medications impact society's health and health care for decades after first use.
- Constant motivation and strength is necessary for an addict to abstain from substance use, maintain recovery, and adopt healthy lifestyle changes.
- A comparative, descriptive, nonexperimental study of a convenience sample of 74 subjects explored health promotion practices of recovering opiate-dependent drug users and compared them with those of abusing opiate-dependent drug users using the Pender's Health-Promoting Lifestyle Profile II.
- Findings showed that recovering opiate-dependent drug users practiced more health-promoting behaviors in all health promotion areas with significant differences in total and subscales scores when compared with the abusing group.
- Nutrition, physical activity, stress management, spiritual growth, interpersonal relationships, and avoidance of high-risk situations are essential health-promoting and relapse-prevention behaviors that recovering individuals need to maintain a healthy lifestyle.

Substance abuse interferes with a person's life purpose and interpersonal relationships. Health care researchers expect that the overuse of alcohol and illicit medications will have an impact on society's health for decades. Many grave physiologic processes can be affected by drug abuse.[1,2] Some of these effects occur when drugs are used at high doses, prolonged use even at the time of the initial dose.

To maintain recovery, addicts must resist the use of mood-altering substances, return to a healthy physical state, repair interpersonal relationships, and develop some sense of peace or spirituality. To accomplish this, substance abusers move through a process in which decisions are made to not only initiate the behavior change but also maintain it.[3,4] No previous studies have focused on opiate-dependent drug users' health behaviors, triggers for relapse, or the changes recovering opiate-dependent

Author has nothing to disclose.
[a] Graduate Nursing, Felician College, 262 South Main Street, Lodi, NJ 07644, USA; [b] Virtua Atlantic Shore Family Practice, 1423 Tilton Road, Northfield, NJ 08225, USA
* 14 Avalon Woods Court, Swainton, NJ 08210-1450.
E-mail address: bradburygolas@comcast.net

drug abusers made in their lives to decrease the incidence of relapse and thereby maintain a healthy, productive lifestyle. Once recovering opiate-dependent drug abusers have not used drugs, do they practice healthy lifestyle behaviors? If so, how do these health-promoting practices/behaviors compare with those of the relapsing opiate-dependent drug user?

Almost 2 million Americans have experimented with heroin, and national trends indicate yearly increases in prescription opiate use.[5] A recent report estimates that 30 million people have used prescription pain relievers, such as oxycodone (OxyContin) and hydrocodone (Vicodin), for nonmedical reasons.[6] As a person continues opiate use over a long period, the body changes and creates powerful cravings that impede the ability to stop using the drugs without intervention. Merely a quick injection, sniff, smoke, or swallow is needed to achieve bliss.[6]

Continued drug use leads to poor prenatal care and an increased number of emergency room visits, including for treatment of abscesses, cellulitis, myocardial infarction, and stroke.[7,8] The user's obsession with substance use disrupts family life and creates a destructive pattern of a codependency, wherein family members supply the user with money to purchase the substance, often denying the problem. Employed drug abusers are more likely to have occupational accidents, affecting either themselves or others.[9]

Addiction is a chronically relapsing disease. In 2002 Gossop and colleagues[10] found that 60% of heroin addicts used heroin within 3 days after treatment. Other studies have shown that heavily using addicts relapse 50% of the time to brief lapses occurring 90% of the time.[11]

Once addicted patients focus on recovery, difficult and extensive lifestyle changes are necessary. Substance abstinence requires constant motivation and strength to maintain recovery. This study was designed to explore the health-promotion practices of recovering opiate-dependent drug users and how they compare with those of abusing opiate-dependent drug users.

LITERATURE REVIEW

Research about substance abuse and relapse has been published in the literature since the 1970s. Studies have shown that 16% to 43% of opiate addicts experience multiple overdoses or die from suicide; only approximately 20% of addicts succeed in recovery.[12-14] Readiness for treatment was shown to be an important factor in predicting treatment retention, participation, and engagement.[15] Expanding on the maturation theory, subsequent studies have shown that recovering addicts begin the formation of a new sense of self, self-identity, and empowerment while in behavioral-cognitive and experiential group therapy.[16,17]

Internal motivation and recovery engagement were shown to be major determinants of relapse prevention. Zeldman and colleagues[18] and Brown[19] showed that female substance abusers who were not fully engaged in the recovery process and who were focused externally participated in more high-risk behaviors than those who were internally focused. Internally motivated participants had lower relapse rates and higher self-efficacy, as evidenced by fewer positive urine samples and better program attendance than externally motivated users.

Much of the early research regarding health and illness used theoretical models that primarily centered on illness prevention, not health promotion. In 1959, Dunn[20] pioneered high-level wellness and health behavior in research and stimulated Pender's[21] development of the Health Promotion Model in the 1980s. Only 2 research studies have explored health promotion and drug users.

Branagan[22] evaluated a nurse-led education program on preventing overdose among 23 methadone treatment clinics in Ireland. Eighty-one percent of the participants responded positively to the educational program, with 71% indicating that they would make changes in their lifestyles based on what they read. Branagan also recommended that the information be distributed to other agencies that have contact with drug users. The study showed a positive response to the education; however, it did not indicate any statistics on overdose knowledge before the education program.

Brondani and Park[23] reviewed the oral health manifestations of patients in methadone maintenance therapy (MMT) and its implications for oral care and primary care/ addiction specialist providers. Methadone use not only is a harm-reduction method for opiate abuse but also decreases the financial burden on the health care system. However, Brondani and Park[23] found that patients on MMT suffered from excessive bacterial plaque accumulation, multiple caries, and serious oral diseases from side effects such as xerostomia, increased sugar craving, and analgesic effects. The authors emphasized the importance of interprofessional care, which includes proper oral hygiene to prevent health-related disorders such as streptococcal infections.

Because of the lack of research on opiate addiction, the literature on nicotine addiction was explored. Tobacco smoking correlates closely with other addictive habits, because research has shown that smoking increases mortality from other health-related illnesses and increases the number of risky lifestyle practices.[24,25] The directional relationship between increased self-efficacy and health-promoting behaviors, specifically not smoking, was predominant in the studies reviewed. Positive relationships between self-efficacy and not initiating smoking, not increasing smoking, and environmental tobacco avoidance were evidenced by Martinelli[26,27] and Kawabata and colleagues.[28] McCleary-Jones[29] found that age, educational level, and income modified health promoting practices in her study of 113 smoking and nonsmoking black women. This study found that educational level is the strongest predictor of practicing health promotion, a finding consistent with that of other studies.[30,31]

Recently studies have examined common medical problems in patients who are recovering from chemical dependency. Alba and colleagues[32] found that chemically dependent individuals without primary care experienced increased hospitalization, reported chronic medical conditions, and practiced unhealthy lifestyle choices. Friedmann and colleagues[33] found that the availability of primary care services at on-site substance treatment programs significantly improved addiction severity at follow-up by 14% but did not change the severity of medical outcome.

Based on the lack of research on health-promoting behaviors during recovery, a study in 2007 explored the health promotion practices of recovering opiate-dependent drug users and how these compared with those of abusing opiate-dependent drug users.

THEORETICAL MODEL

The study was based on Pender's revised health promotion model, which combines numerous constructs from expectancy-value and social cognitive theories within a nursing holistic perspective.[32] The model proposes a positive and humanistic definition of health, and though disease is present, it is not the most important element. Once people commit to a behavior change, their response to the behavior increases their self-efficacy, which in turn increases their likelihood of enacting the behavior. As the person attains substance abstinence, the confidence to maintain the behavior increases, which in turn provides the strength to continue the recovery. The model also proposes that as self-efficacy increases, the number of perceived barriers (eg, loss of a high, withdrawal symptoms) to a specific health behavior decreases. However, in the end, if addicted drug users do not believe that they can succeed at quitting, they will experience relapse and continue to use. The framework for this study's adopted elements of the health promotion model is summarized in **Fig. 1**.

STUDY DESIGN AND MEASURES

A comparative descriptive, exploratory, nonexperimental design was used in this study. A convenience sample of recovering and abusing opiate-dependent drug users from Southern New Jersey was obtained. In addition, for the recovering opiate-dependent drug user sample, snowball sampling was used to achieve an adequate sample size. The abusing opiate-dependent subjects were obtained from a 62-bed, licensed, Joint Commission–accredited addiction treatment center in Southern New Jersey and private outpatient addiction treatment practices. The recovering opiate-dependent drug users were counselors at the inpatient facility or private outpatient practices or were people within the community who attended ongoing outpatient relapse prevention programs. Both groups participated in some form of group therapy, neither of which followed the 12-step program of Narcotics Anonymous. No member of either group was legally obligated to participate in addiction interventions and all were 18 years of age or older. The group facilitators for the inpatient treatment center were predominantly recovering abusers, whereas the facilitators for the outpatient groups possessed education in social work and or psychotherapy.

The dependent variable studied was health promotion practices, specifically those of health responsibility, interpersonal relations, stress management, and spiritual growth, and were measured using the Health-Promoting Lifestyle Profile (HPLP) II.[34] The independent variables in this study were abusing and recovering opiate-dependent drug users, and there were compared.

The demographic data and personal information form was designed by the researcher to describe the abusing and recovering opiate-dependent drug users. Items on the data form are summarized in (**Box 1**). In addition, questions about the number of years recovered and use of any recovery medications were added to the data form for the recovering opiate-dependent drug user.

The HPLP was designed by Walker and colleagues[35] in 1987 to measure current health-promoting practices. The HPLP II measures current health-promoting behaviors using a 52-item, 4-point scale that contains the 6 subscales of nutrition, physical activity, health responsibility, spiritual growth, stress management, and interpersonal relations. Questions concentrate on areas such as time spent with friends and relatives, intake of appropriate foods and servings based on the food pyramid, and time taken for relaxation.

Items are scored on a scale of 1 to 4 (1 = never; 2 = sometimes; 3 = often; 4 = routinely). A composite score and individual subscale scores are obtained through calculating a mean of the responses. The use of means rather than sums of scale items is recommended to retain the 1 to 4 metric of item responses and to allow meaningful comparisons of scores across subscales.[34] Validity and reliability of the tool were previously established. Earlier studies of the HPLP determined content validity through positive correlation with other tools, such as the Personal Lifestyle Questionnaire. Internal reliability of the total HPLP II was reported with a Cronbach alpha score of 0.943. Alphas for each of the subscales range from 0.79 to 0.87 and are as follows: nutrition (0.800), physical activity (0.850), health responsibility (0.861), spiritual growth (0.864), stress management (0.793), and interpersonal relations (0.872).[34]

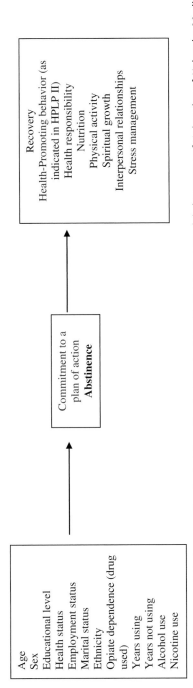

Fig. 1. Theoretical diagram of study concepts adopted from Pender's Revised Health Promotion Model. (*Courtesy of* University of Nebraska Medical Center College of Nursing; with permission.)

> **Box 1**
> **Demographic data and personal information for all subjects**
>
> Age
>
> Educational status and years attended
>
> Marital status
>
> Alcohol use
>
> Number of years using
>
> Weight gain/loss
>
> Sex
>
> Employment status
>
> Ethnicity
>
> Nicotine use
>
> Primary drug used
>
> Health status and problems

PROCEDURE

Once Institutional Review Board approval was granted from the practice and educational facilities, the researcher explained the study to the site counselors and facility research assistants. A standard script was used to explain the study, and the research packets, which included the demographic data and personal information form, HPLP II, and informed consent, were made available at each facility.

On a weekly basis, newly admitted potential subjects were identified and the researcher was notified. A private room was established at both the inpatient and outpatient facilities for the informed consent process. If the participant agreed to complete the study, informed consent was reviewed with each potential participant before survey completion. Voluntary completion of the questionnaires was considered informed consent to participate in the study to ensure participant confidentiality. Persons who did not wish to participate after this explanation were free to leave. Each participant who completed the study then received a $5.00 gift card to a local convenience store.

For the recovering opiate-dependent drug user subjects, the researcher approached the potential participants at a private staff meeting, where management was not present (inpatient facility), or through outpatient patient addiction treatment practice referral or at community outreach prevention programs with permission. The researcher used the same procedure as previously described, beginning with the explanation of the study.

DATA ANALYSIS

The researcher input data collected from the instruments into a computer for analysis using the Statistical Package for the Social Sciences (SPSS/WIN) Version 15.0 for Windows. Descriptive statistics, frequencies, means, ranges, and percentages were used to describe the sample demographic characteristics of each group of opiate-dependent drug users. Chi-square tests were performed to compare the demographic characteristics of the groups. Health-promoting behaviors and practices were measured using the HPLP II. A 1-tailed independent *t* test was used to analyze the total and subscale HPLP II scores of both groups.

RESULTS

A total of 79 abusing and recovering opiate-dependent drug users completed the demographic data form and HPLP II from July through October 2007. Five of these were excluded because of packets that were missing demographic data sheets, leaving 74 total participants.

The demographic and personal characteristics of both the abusing and recovering opiate-dependent drug user groups are shown in **Table 1**. Both groups were predominantly Caucasian with a mean age between 33 and 36 years. The average participant was at least a high school graduate in both groups; however, the recovering group had a higher percentage of college education. Most were either employed full or part time, although the abusing group had a higher percentage of unemployment. The recovering group was evenly split between men and women, whereas the abusing group had a higher percentage of male participants.

The personal health status characteristics of the recovering group differed from those of the abusing group based on several reported parameters, although no significant difference was seen in their personal perception of their overall health. Of the

Table 1
Demographic characteristics of abusing and recovering opiate-dependent drug users

	Abusing (n)	Recovering (n)
Sex		
Male	23 (62.2%)	18 (48.6%)
Female	14 (37.8%)	19 (51.4%)
Marital status		
Single, never married	21 (56.8%)	16 (43.2%)
Married	9 (24.3%)	15 (40.5%)
Divorced/separated	6 (16.2%)	6 (16.2%)
Widowed	1 (2.7%)	—
Current employment status		
Employed, full or part time	18 (48.6%)	25 (67.6%)
Student, full or part time	2 (5.4%)	—
Unemployed	16 (43.2%)	10 (27%)
Retired	1 (2.7%)	2 (5.4%)
Ethnicity		
African American	4 (10.8%)	—
Caucasian/White	33 (89.2%)	36 (97.3%)
Hispanic	—	1 (2.7%)
Education completed		
Grade school only or some high school	7 (18.9%)	5 (13.5%)
High school graduate	18 (48.6%)	15 (40.5%)
Technical school graduate	1 (2.7%)	—
Some college	8 (21.6%)	5 (13.5%)
Associate/baccalaureate degree graduate	3 (8.1%)	11 (29.7%)
Masters/professional degree graduate	—	1 (2.7%)

recovering participants, 97% stated their health to be fair to excellent, compared with 92% of the abusing participants. Years of use were also similar for the groups, averaging between 9 and 10 years, and heroin was the primary drug used (60%–75%). A higher use of oxycodone HCL (OxyContin) was noted in the recovering opiate-dependent group compared with the abusing opiate-dependent group (24% vs 11%, respectively). The use of other drugs in conjunction with the primary agent was markedly higher in the abusing group compared with the recovering group (78% and 54%, respectively). **Table 2** summarizes these differences.

The purpose of this study was twofold, and descriptive and quantitative statistics were used to answer the 2 proposed research questions.

Research Question #1: What Are the Health Promotion Practices of Recovering Opiate-Dependent Drug Users?

Descriptive analysis of the means for the HPLP II (total and 6 subscales) was completed and is summarized in **Table 3**. The mean total score of the HPLP II for the recovering opiate-dependent group reported was 2.78 (standard deviation [SD], 0.563; range, 1.54–4.0) out of a possible score of 4.0. The mean scores for the 6 health promotion subscales ranged from 2.43 to 3.23 out of a possible score of 4.0. These individual means were spiritual growth, 3.23 (SD, 0.565); interpersonal relationships, 3.20 (SD, 0.601); health responsibility, 2.64 (SD, 0.732); nutrition, 2.58 (SD, 0.746); physical activity, 2.43 (SD, 0.863); and stress management, 2.77 (SD, 0.712). The subscales of physical activity and nutrition scored the lowest.

Table 2
Comparison of health characteristics of abusing and recovering opiate-dependent drug users

	Abusing (n)	Recovering (n)
Smoking status		
No	2 (5.4%)	14 (37.8%)
Yes	35 (94.6%)	23 (62.2%)
Current health perception		
Excellent	1 (2.7%)	7 (18.9%)
Good	18 (48.6%)	19 (51.4%)
Fair	15 (40.5%)	10 (27%)
Poor	3 (8.1%)	1 (2.7%)
Drug of choice used		
Heroin	28 (75.7%)	22 (59.5%)
Morphine	1 (2.7%)	1 (2.7%)
Hydrocodone	1 (2.7%)	1 (2.7%)
Oxycodone	2 (5.4%)	3 (8.1%)
Oxycodone HCl	4 (10.8%)	9 (24.3%)
Fentanyl	1 (2.7%)	1 (2.7%)
Use of other types of drugs		
No	8 (21.6%)	17 (45.9%)
Yes	29 (78.4%)	20 (54.1%)
Weight loss/gain of 15 lb in past year		
No	18 (48.6%)	17 (45.9%)
Yes	19 (51.4%)	20 (54.1%)

Table 3
t Test comparison of the Health-Promoting Lifestyle Profile II of abusing and recovering opiate-dependent drug users

Item	Abusing n = 37 M (SD)	Recovering n = 37 M (SD)
Health-promoting behaviors (total)	1.85 (0.412)	2.78 (0.563)[a]
Lifestyle profile subscales		
Health responsibility	1.90 (0.419)	2.64 (0.732)[a]
Physical activity	1.57 (0.537)	2.43 (0.863)[a]
Nutrition	1.66 (0.413)	2.58 (0.746)[a]
Spiritual growth	2.06 (0.611)	3.23 (0.565)[a]
Interpersonal relationships	2.22 (0.679)	3.20 (0.601)[a]
Stress management	1.89 (0.510)	2.77 (0.712)[a]

Abbreviations: M, mean; SD, standard deviation.
[a] Mean group differences were significant at an alpha level; $P<.001$.

Research Question #2: What Are the Differences Between These Health Promotion Practices and Those of Abusing Opiate-Dependent Drug Users?

An independent *t* test analysis was performed to assess differences between the abusing and recovering groups. A significant difference was seen between the groups in the total HPLP score [$t(72) = -8.026$, $P<.001$], indicating that the recovering opiate-dependent drug users practice better health-promoting behaviors than the abusing participants.

In addition, a significant difference was seen in 6 subscale scores of the HPLP II. However, the areas of health responsibility [$t(57.33) = -5.384$, $P<.001$], nutrition [$t(56.2) = -6.752$, $P<.001$], physical activity [$t(60.28) = -5.136$, $P<.001$], and stress management [$t(65.24) = -6.122$, $P<.001$] showed more variability and higher significant mean scores in the recovering group than the abusing group. Although a significant difference was seen between the mean scores of spiritual growth [$t(72) = -8.586$, $P<.001$] and interpersonal relationships [$t(72) = -6.604$, $P<.001$], results showed less variability between the groups (see **Table 3**).

Responses for both groups were normally distributed. Skewed distribution results ranged from 2 to -2 and kurtosis results ranged from 8 to -8. This result indicated a symmetric distribution, which did not interfere with the validity of the *t* test analysis.

DISCUSSION

The average HPLP II score for the recovering opiate-dependent group was 2.78, which was consistent with the range reported by Walker and colleagues.[34] Because no previous studies were found that described this specific vulnerable population, studies with other addictive sample groups were compared. Nies and colleagues[36] found that obese black women performed fewer health-promoting behaviors than nonobese black women. However, no significant difference was seen in the European American sample groups, with an average HPLP score of 2.74. In Wilson's[37] study of homeless women, another vulnerable population, the average HPLP II score was 2.44, which is lower than that found in the present study. In addition, Waite and colleagues[38] found a total HPLP II score of 2.63 in their study of a fitness company workforce. The total HPLP II score for the recovering opiate-dependent group in the present study was similar to that of both general and vulnerable population groups.

Nutrition and physical activity were the lowest subscale scores on the HPLP II. This finding is consistent with that of other studies, with physical activity always scoring lower than nutrition.[36,37,39,40] The recovering opiate-dependent drug users scored lower in the knowledge and implementation of good nutritional habits. Without encouragement from the researcher, several recovering opiate-dependent drug users expressed interest in having an educational seminar on proper nutrition offered during a support group session to improve their eating behaviors.

Health-related personal data showed that the recovering opiate-dependent drug users reported an addiction to oxycodone hydrochloride (OxyContin) more frequently than the abusing group. Only 8% drank alcohol. They continued to smoke tobacco 62% of the time, which is much higher than the 19% reported within the general US population.[41] This percentage is slightly lower than the national average, wherein 70% of those who use drugs also smoke tobacco. Many of this population are unable to relinquish all addictive agents at one time. Most use some form of pharmacologic therapy during recovery.[42–44]

The abusing group's total HPLP II score is significantly lower than what has been reported in the literature when compared with other populations studied. The recovering opiate-dependent drug users scored higher in all subscales of health responsibility, nutrition, physical activity, stress management, spiritual growth, and interpersonal relationships than the abusing group. The higher HPLP II scores reflect that the recovering opiate-dependent drug users were cognizant that positive behaviors can impact their health.

The areas of health responsibility, nutrition, physical activity, and stress management reflected more variability and higher significant mean scores for the recovering group than the abusing group. Although a significant difference was seen between the mean score of spiritual growth and interpersonal relationships, results showed less variability between the groups. This lesser variability cannot be explained, because relapse prevention and recovery programs emphasize positive coping mechanisms to handle stressful, high-risk situations, and self-efficacy–enhancing strategies as a means to prevent relapse, which in turn helps improve these 2 health-promoting behaviors.[42] However, the participants were at varying phases of recovery, ranging from 1 to 10 years. The beginning phases of the recovery process emphasize high-risk avoidance and handling stress; the later phases move toward repairing interpersonal relationships and personal growth. Because participants' nutrition and physical activity scores in both groups were relatively low, programs to improve nutritional and exercise behaviors of both groups are needed.

Relapse prevention programs emphasize the maintenance of new behaviors, which involve avoiding high-risk situations, obtaining increased emotional support, and dealing with life positively. This strategy helps improve self-esteem and increase self-efficacy. This study showed significant differences in health-promoting behaviors between individuals who maintain recovery and those who abuse. Once one begins and maintains the recovery process, the individual can potentially move forward toward a healthier lifestyle. The abusing opiate-dependent drug users' lower scores indicate poorer health practices, which can impact the general biopsychosocial well-being of the person, making them more prone to potential complications and less likely to attempt the recovery process.

Limitations

The study selection limits the results in this study; participants in this study were from only one region from the single state of New Jersey. There was a high percentage of only one ethnic group, which is not representative of the ethnic diversity of the opiate-dependent population in New Jersey at large. Drug-Rehab.org reported that 53.6% of the heroin addicts in New Jersey were white and 39.4% were African American, with the remainder comprising all other ethnicities.[45] In addition, the demographic data and personal characteristic instrument did not contain an item on socioeconomic status, only employment data. An additional methodologic limitation is the lack of sample representation by non–English-speaking participants; this limits the generalizability of this study.

Another limitation was the use of convenience sampling and snowball sampling. Snowball sampling introduces bias by reducing the likelihood that the sample is representative of a cross section from the population. Self reporting by recovering participants as to whether they had not used any substance or had not relapsed in 1 year or longer created a threat to the external validity of the study.

RECOMMENDATIONS

Health promotion practices have been explored in many other vulnerable populations. Developing plans to help people stay healthy and optimize health even in the presence of chronic disease or disability is recognized globally as a major goal for the health care community. Primary health care providers such as physicians, nurse practitioners, and physician assistants can expand their roles to raise health awareness, provide information, encourage decision making, and assist attitudinal, physical, social, and behavioral change in collaboration with their patients.[46] *Healthy People 2010*[47] proposed that opioid-dependent patients be able to receive treatment services and opiate antagonist medication (buprenorphine) in outpatient primary care settings. These services could also include an emphasis on health promotion activities. *Healthy People 2020*[48] proposed multiple new objectives concentrating on reducing and preventing substance use within the adolescent population, thereby possibly decreasing the future incidence of substance abuse in the adult population.

Patients with substance abuse issues are returning to primary care follow-up sooner than the expected 90 days. Because of insurance restrictions, specialty addiction treatment centers no longer keep patients for 28 days; patients are often discharged within 7 days and are expected to be monitored for continued use and any other comorbid conditions by primary care providers. Because of this, primary care health providers are required to know when to contact the addiction specialist or mental health care provider, assess the patient for signs of abuse or adherence to the recovery plan, monitor for adverse effects of addiction-focused pharmacotherapy, and consistently offer support to maintain abstinence. Based on the results of this study, it seems imperative that all health care providers work with patients toward having them become more engaged in their own health.

In the United States, more than 13,000 specialized drug treatment facilities provide counseling, behavioral therapy, medication, case management, and other types of services to persons with substance use disorders.[49] Many of them promote a diet that is high in protein and carbohydrates and low in sugar and caffeine, which helps decrease drug/alcohol cravings and mood swings and rebuild any damaged tissues and organs. Regular physical activity helps ground clients in sobriety and increases endorphins, which help produce a natural drug-free "high" in the brain. It also serves as a vehicle for daily stress release and becomes a safeguard against relapse. Both of these health-promoting activities work toward developing a healthier individual, even if substance use is not present.

Abramsohn and colleagues[50] showed that having a high sense of coherence, in addition to methadone maintenance treatment for opiate addiction, was associated with a higher drug abstinence rate and more successful recovery process. A sense of coherence is based on the development of motivation for coping, belief that stress events are comprehensive, and belief in one's ability to manage the stressful situation. Therefore, patients who have a strong sense of coherence coped with changes and stressors more productively. This concept is something that health care providers should foster in the recovering patient.

Stress management techniques, as part of health promotion, can help opiate-dependent drug users avoid abuse lapses and improve their interpersonal communication skills. These interventions create a circle of positive outcomes, thereby leading to a healthier lifestyle, both physiologically and psychosocially. The constant fear of relapse creates a high stress environment. Often substance abusers must build a new social network, avoid negative people, change occupations or jobs, or move to an entirely different area to reduce stress. Recovering addicts must develop a coping plan for when stress is at its highest so they do not return to bad behaviors. Strategies may include keeping a journal, contacting members of a support team, crying, listening to music, and creating a positive reward system. As recovery progresses and the opiate-dependent drug user improves adherence to health promotion activities, self-esteem and motivation increase to maintain recovery and health.

Pajusco and colleagues[42] found that 97% of heroin addicts were also addicted to nicotine. Many recovery treatment centers prefer not to deal with smoking cessation until a user has first rehabilitated from the substance addiction. However, patients undergoing substance abuse treatment often die of tobacco-related diseases. Although smoking cessation interventions, both behavioral and pharmacologic, ideally should begin in recovery facilities, this treatment most likely begins after addiction treatment and with the primary care provider, adding to the stress a recovering addict experiences after being in the controlled treatment center environment.

Currently the US evidence-based guidelines for "persons with active substance use presenting in primary care" recommend precise screening for substance abuse or dependence, assessment of potential for self-harm, physiologic stabilization, and negotiation with the patient for referral to an addiction specialist.[43] Psychological and mental health issues in primary care physician and nurse practitioner education are usually limited, centering predominantly on depression and anxiety.

With expanded education on care of the addicted patient and strategies that will prevent harm and foster health-promoting behaviors, primary care providers can be provided with the opportunity to successfully intervene with individuals and families dealing with addictions. Screening for dependence, offering counseling, providing education on high-risk events, and teaching skills to cope with high-risk situations, along with pharmacotherapy, may help effect change and help addicted individuals avoid relapses and maintain recovery. In addition, the results of this study support the adoption of health-promoting behaviors.

Patient care is affected by health care policy. Policy determines who gets what kind of care from whom and when.[51] A major role of health care providers is to recognize the needs of the patient and work toward attaining the resources required to provide high-quality patient care. Caring for the addicted and recovering patient in the outpatient primary care setting was a goal of *Health People 2010*,[47] but was not reached. These underserved and misunderstood patients are often treated negatively and inconsistently compared with those with other widely publicized medical conditions, such as cardiovascular and pulmonary disease. Sheridan and colleagues[52] found that 20.8% of drug users reported having treatment refused by dentists compared with 1.6% of nonusers.

The results from this study demonstrate that recovering opiate-dependent drug users adopt better health-promoting behaviors than the abusing population. With better health promotion, health care costs could potentially decrease in future years. In addition, earlier initiation of health promotion in the abusing population may help those individuals avoid major disease complications and assist in substance abuse recovery. However, the initiation of health promotion education and services is not often covered under insurance or Medicaid. Obtaining the financial resources for this endeavor would necessitate creating or changing policy at the insurance company, state, or federal level. Health care providers are empowered to make these changes occur. Grassroots lobbying efforts from the local to federal level enable these policies to come to fruition.

SUMMARY

The results from this study show that recovering opiate-dependent drug users adopt other health-promoting behaviors, such as spiritual growth, health responsibility, and strengthening interpersonal relationships, as they maintain recovery. A significant difference in all health-promoting behaviors is seen between recovering and abusing opiate-dependent drug users. Relapse-prevention therapy, along with other adjunctive treatments to decrease stress, depression, and physical symptoms, increase the addicted person's emotional and spiritual states, energy level, and overall well-being.[53] Primary care providers are at the forefront to successfully intervene with individuals experiencing opiate dependence. With the increase in rapid 3-day addiction detoxification programs in health care institutions, individuals will be relying on primary care practitioners to address their addiction and other health needs.

REFERENCES

1. National Institute for Drug Abuse. Major consequences of drug abuse. Available at: http://nida.nih.gov/consequences/. Accessed October 8, 2012.
2. Miller WR, Rollnick S. Motivational interviewing: preparing people to change addictive behaviors. New York: Gilford Press; 1991.
3. Bandura A. Social foundations of thought and action: a social cognitive theory. Englewood Cliffs (NJ): Prentice Hall; 1986.
4. Ritter AJ. Naltrexone in the treatment of heroin dependence: relationship with depression and risk of overdose. Aust N Z J Psychiatry 2002;36:224–8.
5. McCabe S. Rapid detox: understanding new treatment approaches for the addicted patient. Perspect Psychiatr Care 2001;36(4):113–20.
6. Society for Neuroscience. Treating opiate addiction. Available at: http://www.sfn.org/index.cfm?pagename=brainBriefings_opiateAddiction&print=on. Accessed October 12, 2012.
7. National Institute on Drug Abuse. Addiction science: from molecules to managed care. Available at: www.nida.nih.gov/infofacts/costs.html. Accessed October 12, 2012.
8. National Institute on Drug Abuse. DrugFacts: Drug-related hospital emergency room visits. Available at: www.nida.nih.gov/infofacts/hospitalvisits.html. Accessed October 9, 2012.
9. National Institute on Drug Abuse. DrugFacts: Workplace resources. Available at: www.nida.nih.gov/infofacts/workplace.html. Accessed October 9, 2012.
10. Gossop M, Stewart D, Browne N, et al. Factors associated with abstinence, lapse or relapse to heroin use after residential treatment: protective effect of coping responses. Addiction 2002;97:1259–67.

11. Buddy T. Addiction relapse similar to other chronic diseases. Available at: http://alcoholism.about.com/cs/relapse/a/blcaron030804.htm. Accessed June 3, 2013.
12. Hickman M, Carnwath Z, Madden P, et al. Drug related mortality and fatal overdose risk: pilot cohort study of heroin users recruited from specialist drug treatment sits in London. J Urban Health 2003;80:274–87.
13. Pfab R, Eyer F, Jetzinger E, et al. Cause and motivation in cases of non-fatal drug overdoses in opiate addicts. Clin Toxicol 2006;44:255–9.
14. Galai N, Safaeian M, Vlahov D, et al. Longitudinal patterns of drug injection behavior in the ALIVE study cohort, 1988-2000: description and determinants. Am J Epidemiol 2003;158(7):695–704.
15. Davey-Rothwell M, Frydl A, Latkin C. Does taking steps to control one's drug use predict entry into treatment? Am J Drug Alcohol Abuse 2009;35:279–83.
16. McIntosh J, McKeganey N. Addicts narratives of recovery from drug use: constructing a non-addict identity. Soc Sci Med 2000;50(10):1501–10.
17. Washington O. Using brief therapeutic interventions to create change in self-efficacy and personal control of chemically dependent women. Arch Psychiatr Nurs 2001;XV(1):32–40.
18. Zeldman A, Ryan R, Fiscella K. Motivation, autonomy support, and entity beliefs: their role in methadone maintenance treatment. J Soc Clin Psychol 2004;23(5):675–96.
19. Brown N. Relapsing, running and relieving: a model for high-risk behavior in recovery. J Addict Nurs 2003;14:14–7.
20. Dunn J. What high level wellness means. Canadian Journal of Public Health 1959;50(11):447–57.
21. Pender NJ, Murdaugh CL, Parsons MA. Health promotion in nursing practice. 5th edition. Upper Saddle River (NJ): Prentice Hall; 2006.
22. Branagan O. Providing health education on accidental drug overdose. Nurs Times 2006;102(6):32–3.
23. Brondani M, Park P. Methadone and oral health—a brief review. J Dent Hyg 2011;85(2):92–8.
24. U.S. Department of Health and Human Services. Health effects of cigarette smoking. Available at: http://www.cdc.gov/tobacco/data_statistics/fact_sheets/health_effects/effects_cig_smoking/. Accessed October 26, 2012.
25. Perkins K, Rohay J, Meilahn E, et al. Diet, alcohol, and physical activity as a function of smoking status in middle aged women. Health Psychol 1993;12(5):410–5.
26. Martinelli A. An explanatory model of variables influencing health promotion behaviors in smoking and nonsmoking college students. Public Health Nurs 1999;16(4):263–9.
27. Martinelli A. Testing a model of avoiding environmental tobacco smoke in young adults. Image J Nurs Sch 1999;31(3):237–42.
28. Kawabata T, Cross D, Nishioka N, et al. Relationship between self-esteem and smoking behavior among Japanese early adolescents: initial results from a three-year study. J Sch Health 1999;69(7):280–4.
29. McCleary-Jones V. Health promotion practices of smoking and non-smoking black women. ABNF J 1996;7(1):7–10.
30. Lusk S, Kerr M, Ronis D. Health promoting lifestyles of blue-collar, skilled trade, and white collar workers. Nurs Res 1995;44(1):20–4.
31. Foulds J, Gandhi K, Steinberg M, et al. Factors associated with quitting smoking at a tobacco dependence treatment clinic. Am J Health Behav 2006;30(4):400–12.
32. Alba I, Samet J, Saitz R. Burden of medical illness in drug- and alcohol-dependent persons without primary care. Am J Addict 2004;13:33–45.

33. Friedmann P, Zhang Z, Hendrickson J, et al. Effect of primary medical care on addiction and medical severity in substance abuse treatment programs. J Gen Intern Med 2003;18:1–8.
34. Walker S, Sechrist K, Pender N. Health promoting lifestyle profile II. 1995.
35. Walker S, Sechrist K, Pender N. The health-promoting lifestyle profile: development and psychometric characteristics. Nurs Res 1987;36:76–81.
36. Nies M, Buddington C, Cowan G, et al. Comparison of lifestyles among obese and nonobese African American and European American women in the community. Nurs Res 1998;47(4):251–7.
37. Wilson M. Health-promoting behaviors of sheltered homeless women. Community Health 2005;28(1):51–63.
38. Waite P, Hawks S, Gast J. The correlation between spiritual well-being and health behaviors. Am J Health Promot 1999;13(3):159–62.
39. Kim SY, Jeon EY, Sok S, et al. Comparison of health-promoting behaviors of noninstitutionalized and institutionalized older adults in Korea. J Nurs Scholarsh 2006;38(1):31–5.
40. Haddad L, Kane D, Rajacich D, et al. A comparison of health practices of Canadian and Jordanian nursing students. Public Health Nurs 2004;21(1):85–90.
41. Centers for Disease Control. Adult Cigarette Smoking in the United States: Current Estimate, 2011. Available at: http://www.cdc.gov/mmwr/preview/mmwrhtml/mm5644a2.htm. Accessed June 3, 2013.
42. Witkiewitz K, Marlatt GA. Relapse prevention for alcohol and drug problems. Am Psychol 2004;59(4):224–35.
43. Pajusco B, Chiamulera C, Quaglio G, et al. Tobacco addiction and smoking status in heroin addicts under methadone vs. buprenorphine therapy. Int J Environ Res Public Health 2012;9(3):932–42.
44. Handford C, Kahan M, Srivastava A, et al. Buprenophine/naloxone for opioid dependence: Clinical practice guideline. Centre for Addiction and Mental Health, 2010. Avaliable at: http://guideline.gov/content.aspx?id=39351&search=opioid+addiction#Section420. Accessed June 3, 2013.
45. Drug Rehab, New Jersey. Available at: http://www.drug-rehabs.org/New_Jersey-drug-rehab-alcohol-rehabs-program.htm. Accessed October 9, 2012.
46. Robinson S, Hill Y. The health promoting nurse. J Clin Nurs 1998;7:232–8.
47. Healthy People 2010. Available at:http://www.healthypeople.gov/2010/document/html/objectives/01-05.htm. Accessed May 29, 2013.
48. Healthy People 2020. Available at:http://www.healthypeople.gov/2020/topics objectives2020/objectiveslist.aspx?topicId=40. Accessed May 29, 2013.
49. National Institute on Drug Abuse. Principles of drug addiction treatment: a research-based guide. 3rd edition. Available at: http://www.drugabuse.gov/publications/principles-drug-addiction-treatment/drug-addiction-treatment-in-united-states.
50. Abramsohn Y, Peles E, Potik D, et al. Sense of coherence as a stable predictor for methadone maintenance treatment (MMT) outcome. J Psychoactive Drugs 2009;41(3):249–53.
51. Mason D, Leavitt J, Chaffee M. Policy and politics in nursing and health care. Philadelphia: Elsevier; 2007.
52. Sheridan J, Aggleton M, Carson T. Dental health and access to dental treatment: a comparison of drug users and non-drug users attending community pharmacies. Br Dent J 2001;191(8):453–7.
53. Brooks A, Schwartz G, Reece K, et al. The effect of Johrei healing on substance abuse recovery: a pilot study. J Altern Complement Med 2006;12(7):625–31.

Screening, Brief Intervention, and Referral to Treatment
A Need for Educational Reform in Nursing

Dana Murphy-Parker, MS, CRNP, PMHNP-BC

KEYWORDS

- SBIRT • Screening • Brief intervention • Referral • Addictions • Nursing curricula

KEY POINTS

- The impact of addictions in terms of the global burden of disease is a pandemic. The disability-adjusted life years (DALY), the number of years lost because of ill health, disability, or early death, was approximately 4.0% for both alcohol and tobacco, and 0.8% for illicit drugs.
- According to the International Council of Nurses (ICN), there are 13 million registered nurses across the globe. Envision the substantial decrease in DALY if known effective interventions for substance-related disorders were actually practiced by this number of nurses. Nursing care for individuals, families, and communities should be concentrated on from prevention, early identification, intervention, and treatment of substance-related disorders.
- In the United States, nursing leaders in Addictions Education have stated for the past 3 decades that nursing programs, both at the undergraduate and graduate levels, need to have more didactic content and more clinical practicum experience in nursing education programs. Unfortunately, there has been little progress in this area of nursing education over this period of time.
- It is an established fact that addictions is a healthcare disorder. Research validates that the behavioral and medical treatments that are effective for other chronic disorders, such as diabetes, asthma, and hypertension, can be just as effective for alcohol and drug abuse disorders when comparing compliance and relapse rates.
- The Federal government and The Joint Commission are committed to SBIRT (Screening, brief intervention, and referral to treatment). Nurses are ideally positioned to screen, assess, refer, and, at the advanced practice level, treat clients for substance disorders, provided the knowledge and willingness exists to intervene. A vision for nursing education is the achievement of minimal competencies for all nurses, facilitated by incorporation of substance misuse concepts into nursing education.

College of Nursing and Health Professions, Bellet Building, Room #422, 1505 Race Street, Philadelphia, PA 19102, USA
E-mail address: dam355@drexel.edu

Nurs Clin N Am 48 (2013) 485–489
http://dx.doi.org/10.1016/j.cnur.2013.07.001
0029-6465/13/$ – see front matter © 2013 Elsevier Inc. All rights reserved.

nursing.theclinics.com

The Global Burden of Disease, a worldwide collaboration of more than 100 researchers sponsored by the World Health Organization and the World Bank, revolutionized health priority setting when it published the first plausible description of the world's health.[1] Previous to this, no reliable epidemiologic data set identified global priorities for health services and research.

The use of alcohol, tobacco, and illicit drugs produces considerable disease burden.[2] In 2000, the global burden of disease, as measured in disability-adjusted life years (DALY; number of years lost because of ill health, disability, or early death), was approximately 4.0% for both alcohol and tobacco, and 0.8% for illicit drugs. Tobacco use had the highest mortality rate of all substance use categories, especially for older adults, whereas alcohol use affected younger people both in terms of disabilities and mortality. Both alcohol and tobacco outweighed the use of illegal drugs in terms of disease burden.

Envision the substantial decrease in DALY if known effective interventions for substance-related disorders in individuals, families, and communities were actually practiced by the 13 million nurses worldwide.[3]

More than 20 years ago, the International Council of Nurses (ICN) published a toolkit with the message regarding the role of nurses in managing substance abuse.[4] The purpose of the ICN's message at that time was to raise awareness in the global nursing community that the roles of professional registered nurses had long been recognized as necessary in preventing and minimizing health and social consequences of the substance abuse pandemic, and to increase the number of nurses worldwide committed to reducing the enormous morbidity and mortality associated with substance-related abuse. However, despite the huge health care problems and the tremendous economic costs associated with the global burden of disease, the nursing literature supports negligible amounts of substance misuse content within schools of nursing in the more developed countries, such as Australia, the United Kingdom, and the United States.[5–11]

Millions of individuals experience difficulties related to alcohol and drug addiction in the United States.[12] A report from the Schneider Institute for Health Policy, *Substance Abuse: The Nation's Number One Health Problem*,[13] concluded that more deaths, illnesses, and disabilities are caused by substance abuse than any other preventable conditions. The total economic cost of substance abuse in the United States is estimated to be $559 billion, with the consequences of alcohol, tobacco, and illicit drug use costing $185 billion, $193 billion, and $181 billion, respectively.[14] The fastest growing trend in drug abuse is that of prescription drugs. By 2006, prescription opioids were involved in more overdose deaths than heroin and cocaine combined. In 2007, 27,658 unintentional drug overdose deaths occurred in the United States. Drug overdose deaths were second only to motor vehicle crash deaths among leading causes of unintentional injury deaths.[15]

Since the 1980s in the United States, nurse educators have acknowledged the need for alcohol and drug content in undergraduate nursing education curricula.[16–19] Martinez and Murphy-Parker[20] reviewed the literature and found that the existence of alcohol and drug education in nursing schools devoted little attention to either the theoretical or clinical components of substance abuse education. Unfortunately, little has changed in this educational area since 2003. In a paper presented at the International Nurses Society on Addictions 35th Annual Education Conference, Savage and colleagues[21] compared the amount of content related to alcohol and health included in baccalaureate science of nursing curricula versus the findings of the study conducted by Heinemann and Hoffman[6] 22 years prior. The conclusion was that little progress seemed to have occurred regarding the amount of substance-related content hours required, and that this was disproportionate to the magnitude of the problem. In addition, Savage and colleagues found that the content offered only focused on the treatment of substance-related disorders and did not reflect the shift of focus in the field to include the entire continuum of use and prevention across the life span. As an example, it is now understood that adverse health effects include both the drinker and nondrinker (ie, exposure to risky levels of alcohol affects people across the life span). The large number of nurses employed in diverse health care settings in the United States represents a tremendous opportunity for real change to occur if all nurses are educated and positioned to screen and assess patients with alcohol and drug addictions, and to help determine appropriate treatment options. Nurse educators must seriously evaluate the role of nurses in the addictions treatment workforce, and promote the invaluable influence that nursing can have and has had on the quality of care delivered to individuals with substance-related disorders.[22]

The Screening, Brief Intervention, and Referral to Treatment (SBIRT) approach can help. Research shows SBIRT has a major role in reducing the risk for nondependent unhealthy substance use and in referring eligible patients to specialty treatment for substance abuse.[23] "SBIRT is a comprehensive, integrated, public health approach to the delivery of early intervention and treatment services for persons with substance abuse use disorders, as well as those who are at risk of developing these disorders. Primary care centers, hospital emergency rooms, trauma centers and other community settings provide opportunities for early intervention with at-risk substance users before more severe consequences transpire."[24] Screening is quick and assesses the severity of substance use with the goal of identifying the appropriate level of treatment. Brief intervention/motivational interviewing is used to increase insight and awareness for the individual regarding substance use and motivate them toward behavioral change. If appropriate, referral to treatment is provided to those identified as needing more extensive treatment with access to specialty care. In a nurse-led research study, Broyles and colleagues[25] showed acceptability of nurse-delivered SBIRT care among hospitalized patients. Their results showed that when nurses proceed with confidence, sensitivity, and competence, patients are more comfortable in discussing their alcohol use. Having nurses take the lead in practicing SBIRT makes sense, because they are the ones who spend the most time with patients.

In a letter dated November 1, 2012, American Nurses Association President Karen Daley wrote a letter to Albert Rundio Jr, President of the International Nurses Society on Addictions, stating:

Thank you for sharing the International Nurses Society on Addictions' views on the use of the early intervention tool Screening, Brief Intervention, and Referral and Treatment (SBIRT). At its October meeting, the American Nurses Association (ANA) Board of Directors agreed to the adoption of SBIRT as a tool to be used in all clinical settings.[26]

The Federal government is committed to early SBIRT.[27] In February 2011, the Joint Commission approved alcohol, drug, and tobacco screening; brief intervention; and treatment and follow-up performance metrics that would cover nearly all hospital admissions. The Joint Commission published the SBIRT measure specifications in its standards manual in July 2011, and hospitals can choose SBIRT measures as 1 of 4 measure sets approved by the Joint Commission for public reporting.[28]

The time has come to raise awareness within the entire nursing community that it is no longer acceptable for health care professionals to think of substance abuse and substance dependence as a matter of patients being morally deficient or lacking the willpower to quit. It is not a "just say no" problem. Research validates that the behavioral and medical treatments that are effective for other chronic disorders, such as diabetes, asthma, and hypertension, can be just as effective for alcohol and drug abuse disorders when comparing compliance and relapse rates.[29]

With the prevalence of addiction-related health consequences, all nurses must maintain a basic level of knowledge and skills regarding addictions.[30] Nurses are ideally positioned to screen, assess, refer, and, at the advanced practice level, treat clients for substance disorders, provided the knowledge and willingness exists to intervene. A vision for nursing education is the achievement of minimal competencies for all generalist nurses, facilitated by incorporation of substance misuse concepts into nursing education.[31] An urgent need exists to disseminate the most recent knowledge and skills in nursing school curricula throughout the United States and internationally. Evidence in the nursing literature indicates that education is a key predictor of nurses' knowledge and therapeutic attitudes toward patients with substance-related disorders.[32] The integration of substance abuse education into nursing school curricula is long overdue.

REFERENCES

1. Murray CJ, Lopez AD. The global burden of disease: a comprehensive assessment of mortality and disability from disease, injuries and risk factors in 1990 and projected to 2020. Cambridge (MA): Harvard School of Public Health; 1996.
2. Rehm J, Taylor B, Room R. Global burden of disease from alcohol, illicit drugs and tobacco. Drug Alcohol Rev 2006;25(6):503–13.
3. Global Nursing Numbers. Available at: http://www.leamingnurse.org/index.php/library/nurse-numbers. Accessed August 7, 2013.
4. Sheehan A. Nurses respond to substance abuse. Int Nurs Rev 1992;39(5):141–4.
5. Murphy SA. The urgency of substance abuse education in schools of nursing. J Nurs Educ 1989;28(6):248–51.
6. Heinemann ME, Hoffman GL. Nurse educators look at alcohol education for the profession. Alcohol Health Res World 1989;13(1):48–51.
7. Rassool GH, Oyefeso N. The need for substance misuse education in health studies curriculum: a case for nursing education. Nurse Educ Today 1993;13:107–10.
8. Sullivan EJ, Handley SM. Alcohol and drug abuse. In: Fitzpatarick JJ, Stevenson JS, editors. Annual review of nursing research, vol. 11. New York: Springer; 1993. p. 281–9.
9. Naegle MA. Education, research and theory development. In: Sullivan EJ, editor. Nursing care of clients with substance abuse. St Louis (MO): Mosby; 1995. p. 409–21.
10. Sullivan EJ. Nursing care of clients with substance abuse. St Louis (MO): Mosby; 1995.
11. Happell B, Taylor C. Drug and alcohol education for nurses: have we examined the whole problem? J Addict Nurs 1999;11(4):180–5.
12. Murphy-Parker D, Martinez R. Nursing perspective of global substance abuse and misuse: US and UK differences. Drugs and Alcohol Today 2001;1(1):35–42.
13. Schneider Institute for Health Policy. Substance abuse: the nation's number one health problem. Princeton (NJ): Robert Woods Johnson Foundation; 2001.
14. Rundio A. SBIRT – the new 6th vital sign: a policy perspective. J Addict Nurs 2012;23(3):208–9.
15. Unintentional drug poisoning in the United States. Centers for Disease Control and Prevention Web site. Available at: http://www.cdc.gov/HomeandRecreationalSafety/pdf/poison-issue-brief.pdf. Accessed July 25, 2013.

16. Burns EM, Thompson A, Ciccone AJ. An addictions curriculum for nurses and other helping professionals. New York: Springer; 1989.
17. Church M, Fisk NB, Neafsey PJ. Curriculum for nursing education in alcohol and drug abuse. Storrs (CT): University of Connecticut School of Nursing; 1990.
18. Naegle M, editor. Substance abuse education in nursing, vols. 1–3. Binghamton (NY): National League for Nursing; 1991 & 1993.
19. Murray MM, Savage C. The NIAAA BSN nursing education curriculum: a rationale and overview. J Addict Nurs 2010;21(1):3–5.
20. Martinez RJ, Murphy-Parker D. Examining the relationship of addiction education and beliefs of nursing students toward persons with alcohol problems. Arch Psychiatr Nurs 2003;17(4):156–64.
21. Savage C, Dyehouse J, Marcus M, et al. Alcohol and health content in Baccalaureate nursing programs: a 24 year perspective. Presented at the International Nurses Society on Addictions Annual Education Conference. Tucson, September 7–10, 2011.
22. Fornili K. Another quality chasm: the failure of nursing to clearly communicate its role within the addiction treatment workforce. J Addict Nurs 2007;18(1):57–9.
23. Saitz R, Galanter M. Alcohol/drug screening and brief intervention: advances in evidenced based practice. Binghamton (NY): Haworth Medical Press; 2007.
24. Substance Abuse and Mental Health Services Administration. Screening, Brief Intervention, and Referral to Treatment (SBIRT). Available at: http://www.samhsa.gov/prevention/sbirt. Accessed July 25, 2013.
25. Broyles LM, Rosenberger E, Hanusa BH, et al. Hospitalized patients' acceptability of nurse-delivered screening, brief intervention, and referral to treatment. Alcohol Clin Exp Res 2012;36(4):725–31.
26. Daley KA. Letter to International Nurses Society on Addictions to support partnering with the American Nurses Association to promote the use of SBIRT in nursing clinical practice. Silver Springs (MD): American Nurses Association; 2012.
27. Fornili K, Alemi F. Medicaid reimbursement for screening and brief intervention: amending the medicaid state plan and approving state appropriations for the medicaid state match. J Addict Nurs 2007;18(4):225–32.
28. The Joint Commission. Substance use. Available at: http://www.jointcommission.org/substance_use. Accessed July 25, 2013.
29. McLellan AT, Lewis DC, O'Brien CP, et al. Drug dependence, a chronic medical illness: implications for treatment, insurance, and outcomes evaluation. JAMA 2000;284(13):1689–95.
30. American Nurses Association & International Nurses Society on Addictions. Scope and standards of addictions nursing practice. Washington (DC): ANA; 2004.
31. Naegle M. Nursing education in the prevention and treatment of SUD. Subst Abus 2002;23(Suppl 3):247–61.
32. Rassool H. Some considerations on attitudes to addictions: waiting for the tides to change. J Addict Nurs 2007;18(2):61–3.

Index

Note: Page numbers of article titles are in **boldface** type.

Nurs Clin N Am 48 (2013) 491–497
http://dx.doi.org/10.1016/S0029-6465(13)00079-0
0029-6465/13/$ – see front matter © 2013 Elsevier Inc. All rights reserved.

nursing.theclinics.com